Family-Centered Services in Residential Treatment: New Approaches for Group Care

Family-Centered Services in Residential Treatment: New Approaches for Group Care has been co-published simultaneously as *Residential Treatment for Children & Youth,* Volume 17, Number 3 2000.

The *Residential Treatment for Children & Youth* Monographic "Separates"

Below is a list of "separates," which in serials librarianship means a special issue simultaneously published as a special journal issue or double-issue *and* as a "separate" hardbound monograph. (This is a format which we also call a "DocuSerial.")

"Separates" are published because specialized libraries or professionals may wish to purchase a specific thematic issue by itself in a format which can be separately cataloged and shelved, as opposed to purchasing the journal on an on-going basis. Faculty members may also more easily consider a "separate" for classroom adoption.

"Separates" are carefully classified separately with the major book jobbers so that the journal tie-in can be noted on new book order slips to avoid duplicate purchasing.

You may wish to visit Haworth's website at . . .

http://www.haworthpressinc.com

. . . to search our online catalog for complete tables of contents of these separates and related publications.

You may also call 1-800-HAWORTH (outside US/Canada: 607-722-5857), or Fax: 1-800-895-0582 (outside US/Canada: 607-771-0012), or e-mail at:

getinfo@haworthpressinc.com

Family-Centered Services in Residential Treatment: New Approaches for Group Care, edited by John Y. Powell, PhD (Vol. 17, No. 3, 2000). *"Offers suggestions and methods for incorporating parents and youths into successful treatment programs in temporary and long-term settings. This essential guide will help psychologists, therapists, and social workers unite theory and practice to create a family-oriented environment for troubled clients and provide effective services. Containing case studies, personal discoveries, and insights about the potentials and limitations of residential care, this reliable resource will help you develop improved services for youths with the help of their families using reevaluated techniques to meet individual needs."*

The New Board: Changing Issues, Roles and Relationships, edited by Raymon Schimmer, MAT, and Nadia Finkelstein, MS, ACSW (Vol. 16, No. 4, 1999). *This innovative book offers very specific, real life examples and informed recommendations for board management of non-profit residential services agencies and explains why and how to consider redesigning your board form and practice. You will explore variations of board structures, managed care pressure, increased complexity of service, reduced board member availability, and relevant theoretical discussions complete with pertinent reports on the practice of boards in the nonprofit residential field.*

Outcome Assessment in Residential Treatment, edited by Steven I. Pfeiffer, PhD (Vol. 13, No. 4, 1996). *"Presents a logical and systematic response, based on research, to the detractors of residential treatment centers." (Canada's Children (Child Welfare League of Canada))*

Residential Education as an Option for At-Risk Youth, edited by Jerome Beker, EdD, and Douglas Magnuson, MA (Vol. 13, No. 3, 1996). *"As a remarkable leap forward, as an approach to child welfare, it is required reading for professionals–from child care workers to administrators and planners–or for anyone in search of hope for children trapped in the bitter problems of a blighted and disordered existence . . . It is instructive, practical, and humanistic." (Howard Goldstein, DSW, Professor Emeritus, Case Western Reserve University; Author, The Home on Gorham Street)*

When Love Is Not Enough: The Management of Covert Dynamics in Organizations that Treat Children and Adolescents, edited by Donna Piazza, PhD (Vol. 13, No. 1, 1996). *"Addresses the difficult question of 'unconscious dynamics' within institutions which care for children and adolescents. The subject matter makes for fascinating reading, and anyone who has had experience of residential institutions for disturbed children will find themselves nodding in agreement throughout the book." (Emotional and Behavioural Difficulties)*

Applied Research in Residential Treatment, edited by Gordon Northrup, MD (Vol. 12, No. 1, 1995). *"The authors suggest appropriate topics for research projects, give practical suggestions on design, and provide example research reports." (Reference & Research Book News)*

Managing the Residential Treatment Center in Troubled Times, edited by Gordon Northrup, MD (Vol. 11, No. 4, 1994). *"A challenging manual for a challenging decade. . . .Takes the eminently sensible position that our failures are as worthy of analysis as our successes. This approach is both sobering and instructive." (Nancy Woodruff Ment, MSW, BCD, Associate Executive Director, Julia Dyckman Andrus Memorial, Yonkers, New York)*

The Management of Sexuality in Residential Treatment, edited by Gordon Northrup, MD (Vol. 11, No. 2, 1994). *"Must reading for residential treatment center administrators and all treatment personnel." (Irving N. Berlin, MD, Emeritus Professor, School of Medicine, University of New Mexico; Clinical Director, Child & Adolescent Services, Charter Hospital of Albuquerque and Medical Director, Namaste Residential Treatment Center)*

Sexual Abuse and Residential Treatment, edited by Wander de C. Braga, MD, and Raymond Schimmer (Vol. 11, No. 1, 1994). *"Ideas are presented for assisting victims in dealing with past abuse and protecting them from future abuse in the facility." (Coalition Commentary (Illinois Coalition Against Sexual Assault))*

Milieu Therapy: Significant Issues and Innovative Applications, edited by Jerome M. Goldsmith, EdD, and Jacquelyn Sanders, PhD (Vol. 10, No. 3, 1993). *This tribute to Bruno Bettelheim illuminates continuing efforts to further understanding of the caring process and its impact upon healing and repair measures for disturbed children in residential care.*

Severely Disturbed Youngsters and the Parental Alliance, edited by Jacquelyn Sanders, PhD, and Barry L. Childress, MD (Vol. 9, No. 4, 1992). *"Establishes the importance of a therapeutic alliance with the parents of severely disturbed young people to improve the success of counseling." (Public Welfare)*

Crisis Intervention in Residential Treatment: The Clinical Innovations of Fritz Redl, edited by William C. Morse, PhD (Vol. 8, No. 4, 1991). *"Valuable in helping us set directions for continuing Redl's courageous trail-blazing work." (Reading (A Journal of Reviews and Commentary in Mental Health))*

Adolescent Suicide: Recognition, Treatment and Prevention, edited by Barry Garfinkel, MD, and Gordon Northrup, MD (Vol. 7, No. 1, 1990). *"Distills highly relevant information about the identification and treatment of suicidal adolescents into a pithy volume which will be highly accessible by all mental health professionals." (Norman E. Alessi, MD, Director, Child Diagnostic and Research Unit, The University of Michigan Medical Center)*

Psychoanalytic Approaches to the Very Troubled Child: Therapeutic Practice Innovations in Residential and Educational Settings, edited by Jacquelyn Sanders, PhD, and Barry M. Childress, MD (Vol. 6, No. 4, 1989). *"I find myself wanting to re-read the book–which I recommend for every professional library shelf, especially for directors of programs dealing with the management of residentially located disturbed youth." (Journal of American Association of Psychiatric Administrators)*

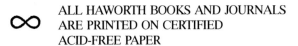

Family-Centered Services in Residential Treatment: New Approaches for Group Care

John Y. Powell, PhD
Editor

Family-Centered Services in Residential Treatment: New Approaches for Group Care has been co-published simultaneously as *Residential Treatment for Children & Youth,* Volume 17, Number 3 2000.

The Haworth Press, Inc.
New York • London • Oxford

Family-Centered Services in Residential Treatment: New Approaches for Group Care has been co-published simultaneously as *Residential Treatment for Children & Youth* ™, Volume 17, Number 3 2000.

The development, preparation, and publication of this work has been undertaken with great care. However, the publisher, employees, editors, and agents of The Haworth Press and all imprints of The Haworth Press, Inc., including The Haworth Medical Press® and Pharmaceutical Products Press®, are not responsible for any errors contained herein or for consequences that may ensue from use of materials or information contained in this work. Opinions expressed by the author(s) are not necessarily those of The Haworth Press, Inc.

Cover design by Thomas J. Mayshock Jr.

Library of Congress Cataloging-in-Publication Data

Family-centered services in residential treatment : new approaches for group care / John Y. Powell, editor.
     p. cm.
     "Co-published simultaneously as Residential treatment for children & youth, volume 17, number 3 2000."
     Includes bibliographical references and index.
     ISBN 0-7890-1021-6 (alk. paper)–ISBN 0-7890-1022-4 (alk. paper)
     1. Children–Institutional care. 2. Social work with children. I. Powell, John Y. II. Residential treatment for children & youth.
HV862 .F36 2000
362.73'2–dc21
                                                         00-038856

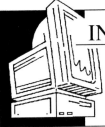

INDEXING & ABSTRACTING

Contributions to this publication are selectively indexed or abstracted in print, electronic, online, or CD-ROM version(s) of the reference tools and information services listed below. This list is current as of the copyright date of this publication. See the end of this section for additional notes.

- *Applied Social Sciences Index & Abstracts (ASSIA) (Online: ASSI via Data-Star) (CDRom: ASSIA Plus)*

- *BUBL Information Service, an Internet-based Information Service for the UK higher education community <URL: http://bubl.ac.uk/>*

- *Cambridge Scientific Abstracts*

- *Child Development Abstracts & Bibliography*

- *CNPIEC Reference Guide: Chinese National Directory of Foreign Periodicals*

- *Criminal Justice Abstracts*

- *Exceptional Child Education Resources (ECER) (CD/ROM from SilverPlatter and hard copy)*

- *Family Studies Database (online and CD/ROM)*

- *IBZ International Bibliography of Periodical Literature*

- *Index to Periodical Articles Related to Law*

- *International Bulletin of Bibliography on Education*

- *Mental Health Abstracts (online through DIALOG)*

- *National Clearinghouse on Child Abuse & Neglect Information*

- *National Criminal Justice Reference Service*

(continued)

- *Psychological Abstracts (PsycINFO)*

- *Sage Family Studies Abstracts (SFSA)*

- *Social Planning/Policy & Development Abstracts (SOPODA)*

- *Social Work Abstracts*

- *Sociological Abstracts (SA) http://www.csa.com*

- *Sociology of Education Abstracts*

- *Special Educational Needs Abstracts*

- *Violence and Abuse Abstracts: A Review of Current Literature on Interpersonal Violence (VAA)*

Special Bibliographic Notes related to special journal issues (separates) and indexing/abstracting:

- indexing/abstracting services in this list will also cover material in any "separate" that is co-published simultaneously with Haworth's special thematic journal issue or DocuSerial. Indexing/abstracting usually covers material at the article/chapter level.

- monographic co-editions are intended for either non-subscribers or libraries which intend to purchase a second copy for their circulating collections.

- monographic co-editions are reported to all jobbers/wholesalers/approval plans. The source journal is listed as the "series" to assist the prevention of duplicate purchasing in the same manner utilized for books-in-series.

- to facilitate user/access services all indexing/abstracting services are encouraged to utilize the co-indexing entry note indicated at the bottom of the first page of each article/chapter/contribution.

- this is intended to assist a library user of any reference tool (whether print, electronic, online, or CD-ROM) to locate the monographic version if the library has purchased this version but not a subscription to the source journal.

- individual articles/chapters in any Haworth publication are also available through the Haworth Document Delivery Service (HDDS).

Family-Centered Services in Residential Treatment: New Approaches for Group Care

CONTENTS

ABOUT THE EDITOR

John Y. Powell, PhD, is Professor of Social Work at East Carolina University, Greenville, NC, and is also Lead Professor of the Child/Family Area of Specialization in the Master of Social Work Program. He is Editor of the Book Review Section and serves on the Editorial Board of *Residential Treatment for Children & Youth.* Prior to his academic appointment, he worked for 24 years in residential treatment–including services as CEO of Hillside in Atlanta, Georgia, and Thompson Children's Home in Charlotte, NC. Long interested in family-centered practice in residential settings, Dr. Powell earned a doctorate in Family Relations from the University of North Carolina-Greensboro. He is licensed as both a Clinical Social Worker and a Marriage & Family Therapist. The NC Association of Marriage & Family Therapists presented him the "Champion of the Family" Award in 1999.

Preface and Tribute

John Y. Powell, PhD

Dedicated in memory and tribute
to the late Alan Keith-Lucas, PhD, 1910-1995

Alan Keith-Lucas served for many years as the Editor of the Book Review Section and on the Editorial Board of *Residential Treatment for Children & Youth*. Throughout his professional career (over more than 50 years) as a practitioner, social work educator, consultant to children's residential agencies, and prolific writer, Keith-Lucas was an advocate for family-centered services. His 1977 book (with Clifford W. Sanford), *Group Child Care as a Family Service*, helped set the stage for today's interest in family-centered services. Dr. Keith-Lucas believed "family-centered" to be a central value that a professional or agency could use to organize practice; he rejected its use as a simplistic, sentimental slogan. His lecture, "Child-Centered or Family-Centered?," although delivered in 1979, continues to be timely, and it is reprinted as the lead article.

It might appear to the casual observer that concepts of family-centered practice have been discovered only recently and are incompatible with residential treatment or longer term group care; but this is not necessarily so. A colleague and leader in residential treatment, Douglas Powers, MD, recorded a project at the Virginia Treatment Center for Children (Medical College of Virginia, Richmond) in the 1960s when interdisciplinary traveling teams from the residential treatment center traversed that state (and still do) to keep alive the ties between hospitalized children and their families and communities (Powers, 1980). Douglas Powers' wonderful

[Haworth co-indexing entry note]: "Preface and Tribute." Powell, John Y. Co-published simultaneously in *Residential Treatment for Children & Youth* (The Haworth Press, Inc.) Vol. 17, No. 3, 2000, pp. xix-xxiii; and: *Family-Centered Services in Residential Treatment: New Approaches for Group Care* (ed: John Y. Powell) The Haworth Press, Inc., 2000, pp. xiii-xvii. Single or multiple copies of this article are available for a fee from The Haworth Document Delivery Service [1-800-342-9678, 9:00 a.m. - 5:00 p.m. (EST). E-mail address: getinfo@haworthpressinc.com].

xiii

poetry also enlivens this special issue; his poetry expands "family-centered" to include viewpoints of placed children.

James Whittaker's contribution, "Reinventing Residential Childcare: An Agenda for Research and Practice," was first delivered at a Duke Endowment sponsored 1997 East Carolina University symposium, "Fresh Thinking about Group Care for Children." In fact, Jim Whittaker's address and the symposium sparked the idea for this special issue. Dr. Whittaker's outstanding and vast contributions to the literature of residential treatment and group care span thirty plus years [including *The Other 23 Hours* (with Trieschman & Brendtro) (Aldine, 1969), *Caring for Troubled Children: Residential Treatment in a Community Context* (Aldine, 1979) to his present article]. No recent convert to family-centered practice, his book *Caring for Troubled Children* includes a chapter "Parents as Partners in Helping." His article in this special issue advises that we move away from polarized thinking and look afresh at both the potential and limitations of residential care.

No "family-centered" volume would be sufficient without the voice of a family member. In the third article, Ms. Sandra Spencer, a parent of a child with a serious emotional disturbance and a professional family advocate, poignantly describes the placement of her son in two residential settings–first in a community-based facility ten minutes from their home and later in a university hospital setting over one hundred miles away. Her reflections demonstrate that "family-centered" practice cannot be achieved by close proximity alone for the nearby agency made contacts difficult whereas the hospital welcomed her visits and set up special times for telephone calls to the attending psychiatrist. Her family's experiences are important to consider.

Since 1924, the Duke Endowment has advanced residential care in North and South Carolina, and their recently sponsored "Carolinas Project" moved "family-centered" from a peripheral to a central concept for many Carolinas children's residential agencies. Dr. Floyd Alwon and colleagues describe agency change and growth in "The Carolinas Project: A Comprehensive Intervention to Support Family-Centered Group Care Practice." Their article is followed by "Joining Family-Centered Care and the Team Approach: A Conversation About the Process," a paper by staff members from the Children's Home, Inc , a Winston-Salem, NC, residential agency that participated in the

Carolinas Project. It demonstrates how theory can be united with practice.

"Questioning the Continuum of Care: Toward a Reconceptualization of Child Welfare Services" by Earl Stuck, Richard Small and Frank Ainsworth calls for an even more comprehensive reappraisal of "family-centered" practice as they question the child welfare system's basic approach to out of home placements. This is followed by "Looking Back to See Ahead" a moving account of "growing up" in an orphanage-oriented residential center by James Campbell who offers personal but informed suggestions for retaining the best from group care's past while finding new and more creative ways to provide longer-term group care. Campbell's recollections and insights are brought into a larger arena by Carol Levine in "AIDS and a New Generation of Orphans: Is There a Role for Group Care?" She points out that thousands of children have been orphaned or will likely soon be orphaned as a result of the AIDS epidemic, and she, as one of this group of children's most important advocates, wonders if group care might be a suitable alternative to provide supplemental parenting for some of these children. In raising this alternative, Ms. Levine has created anxiety in other child/family advocates who fear a retreat to the orphanages of old.

The final article, "Celebrating Change: A Schema for Family-Centered Practice in Residential Settings," by Lessie Bass, David Dosser and John Powell, reports the development and findings of a Duke Endowment funded research project. The authors developed a helping process model that was openly shared with families in two residential agencies to help plot and direct placements. Terms like "diagnosis," "evaluation," and "treatment" were replaced by "discovery," "change," and "celebration." The schema process appears promising, but can residential centers that provide care, beyond short periods of time, break free of their orphanage legacies and reinvent themselves as family-centered agencies?

Is family-centered residential care an oxymoron? Dr. Michael Blackwell, President of the Baptist Children's Homes of NC believes longer term care can indeed be family-centered:

> For many youth, the best permanent plan is for them to live in a long-term residential setting. Relationship needs and developmental issues often can be best met through a peer group setting. Psychological permanency is also crucial, both through meeting

daily physical needs while enabling the youth to maintain an identity and psychological connection with his/her family network. Programs of intentionalized services provide a clear, concise purpose and focus for each service in a continuum of care. Dr. Alan Keith-Lucas, as early as the middle 1970's, promoted the notion of task-focused residential services. Recognizing that residential services needed to move from generalized congregate care to a more specialized, task-centered program, he began to help residential programs recognize the importance of family-focused work.

Reuniting every child and parent is not realistic for all youth; residential programs must establish a partnership with a parent to enable the parent to be as active as possible to assure his or her child of psychological permanency even if long-term residential care is involved. Dr. Keith-Lucas called this "parents as partners" or "supplemental parenting." The intent is that the residential facility will supplement what the parent cannot provide relative to meeting both the youth's daily basic needs, in addition to long-range and identity issues.

The modeling/teaching of parenting skills by an entire service delivery team is one way to equip the parent to better achieve parenting skills. Aggressively involving the parent in the daily life events of the child, such as birthdays, school conferences, participation in special school or campus events, meals in cottage, overnight visits on campuses, further supports the parental role. Parents are valued and recognized as essential partners in the care of their children. The debate should not be "should" and "can" long-term residential service be an option for "today's children and youth," but how can an organization increase its effectiveness in providing psychological permanency for youth in a peer group setting. Institutions shouldn't assume the role of parent, but aggressively be enabling parents and children in long-term care to maintain involvement, identity, and psychological connections. (Personal communication, June 30, 1999)

Family-centered practice is, at its best, a professional value and commitment that drives policy and practice. A serious embrace of family-centered practice, whether by an individual or by an agency, is a somewhat sacred undertaking. It requires what Alan Keith-Lucas referred to as a bold and honest "clarification" process with families which might have various results, such as: (a) reunification of placed children to their nuclear families, (b) assumptions of care by extended family members and friends, (c) releases of children to other families by adoption, and (d) decisions that some children, usually teenagers, might need to grow up living largely in supplemental care apart from their natural or adoptive families–but none-the-less remaining bound to their families. On this latter point, is this much different from some children who "grow up" in boarding schools? When I was serving as the director of a residential treatment-oriented program, a friend who was a headmaster at an expensive preparatory boarding school and I used to compare the reasons for placements at both settings. We concluded that many families with children (especially adolescents) in both settings needed institutional assistance (i.e., supplemental parenting) to successfully rear their children. Ironically, families of children in the expensive boarding school were often praised for their sacrifice, whereas families of children placed in treatment centers or public/ charitable group care were often ridiculed.

Salvador Minuchin (1995) says "the family is at once the best and worst we have. But the worst aspects of the family, and there are many, (have) been very well described. It (is) the strength of the family–the resources and possibilities–that (have) been left utterly unexplored." This Special Issue of *Residential Treatment for Children & Youth* hopefully will help readers to explore family possibilities and rethink family-centered services in residential settings. I thank all the contributors for their timely and meaningful articles and poetry that will assist in that process.

John Y. Powell

REFERENCES

Keith-Lucas, A. (1977) *Group child care as a family service.* Chapel Hill: UNC Press.

Minuchin, S. (1995) Foreword. In P. Adams & K. Nelson's (Eds.), *Reinventing human services.* Hawthorne, NY: Aldine de Gruyter.

Powers, D. (1980) *Creating environments for troubled children.* Chapel Hill: UNC Press.

Trieschman, A.E., Whittaker, J.K. & Brendtro, L.K. (1969) *The other 23 hours: Child care work with emotional disturbed children in a therapeutic milieu.* New York: Aldine de Gruyter.

Whittaker. J.K. (1997) *Caring for troubled children: Residential treatment in a community context* (paperback edition). Hawthorne, NY: Aldine de Gruyter.

"You Never Know"

In the middle of January,
In the midst of a snowstorm
We carefully wedged
The completed birdhouse
Into a high crotch
Of an old cedar tree,
Under his supervision.

He built the birdhouse himself
With utmost care
In woodworking class
And its installation
Could not be delayed
Even though spring was not
Just around the corner

You never know, he said
When some homeless bird
Might stray by
And want to live there
You just never know.

Now we inspect the house
Periodically
From the correct distance
So as not to frighten
A possible occupant.

Dr. Powers may be written at 5517 Eagle Lake Drive South, Charlotte, NC 28217.

[Haworth co-indexing entry note]: "You Never Know." Powers, Douglas. Co-published simultaneously in *Residential Treatment for Children & Youth* (The Haworth Press, Inc.) Vol. 17, No. 3, 2000 , pp. 1-2; and: *Family-Centered Services in Residential Treatment: New Approaches for Group Care* (ed: John Y. Powell) The Haworth Press, Inc., 2000, pp. 1-2. Single or multiple copies of this article are available for a fee from The Haworth Document Delivery Service [1-800-342-9678, 9:00 a.m. - 5:00 p.m. (EST). E-mail address: getinfo@haworthpressinc.com].

But occasionally, nonetheless
He asks to be hoisted
For a closer look.
You never know when, he says,
You just never know.

Douglas Powers, MD

BIOGRAPHICAL NOTE

Douglas Powers is a consulting child-adolescent psychiatrist and Distinguished Professor Emeritus in the College of Education and Allied Professions, The University of North Carolina at Charlotte. He was formerly the Book Review Editor of this journal.

Child-Centered or Family-Centered?

Alan Keith-Lucas, PhD

Although Alan Keith-Lucas died in 1995, his pioneering thoughts about families, children and group care programs live on in the practice of many professionals and agencies, especially in the Southeastern United States. He strongly believed in family-centered services. His address of 1979 is included in this volume as it clearly defines and contrasts "family-centered" and "child-centered" approaches.

Given this title I'd have to say that words are slippery things; that one could quite easily show that to be family-centered is in fact to be child-centered, although the opposite is rather harder to prove. But let me let you in on a secret. This (1979) is the International Year of the Child. As someone whose reputation is that of a friend of children, and I hope that is not wholly undeserved, I might be expected to rejoice that children were getting so much attention. But my first reaction to the Year of the Child was a whispered, "Please, God, no!"

That may take some explanation. Certainly we need to look at the plight of children all over the world, and in our own country too. Compared with many countries, we do not, as a people, value children as we should. Even our neighbor to the South, whom we tend to look on as backward, appears to be more concerned about what happens to

---

Given at the Annual Forum of Thompson Children's Home (Episcopal), Charlotte, NC, 1979.

[Haworth co-indexing entry note]: "Child-Centered or Family-Centered?" Keith-Lucas, Alan. Co-published simultaneously in *Residential Treatment for Children & Youth* (The Haworth Press, Inc.) Vol. 17, No. 3, 2000, pp. 3-9; and: *Family-Centered Services in Residential Treatment: New Approaches for Group Care* (ed: John Y. Powell) The Haworth Press, Inc., 2000, pp. 3-9. Single or multiple copies of this article are available for a fee from The Haworth Document Delivery Service [1-800-342-9678, 9:00 a.m. - 5:00 p.m. (EST). E-mail address: getinfo@haworthpressinc.com].

its children than we can be said to be; and we are certainly behind several European countries in the proportion of our resources that we spend on children's health, their education and indeed their support. We are one of the few industrialized countries without a Children's Allowance plan. The sort of advocacy for children that seeks better living conditions for the families in which most children grow up, that furthers their health and education, is an admirable thing. But it is more than advocacy for children. It is advocacy for family life.

It is advocacy for children apart from their families that scares me. For that kind of advocacy attracts a whole lot of people who are not so much advocates for children as they are adversaries to their parents. These are people who love children, who talk long and loud about children's rights, who think of children as innocent victims of their parents' mistreatment and get very indignant about it, who want to take over and bring up children according to their own ideas. They are not so much child-advocates as parental interveners. They rarely talk with children. They are more inclined to talk down to them. If they did talk with children they might get some unpleasant surprises. Children often resent them bitterly. But instead of talking with children, being true advocates to the sense of doing what children have asked them to do, they just decide what is good for them.

Sometimes, of course they are right. There are some children who do need protection from parents who are so troubled or sick that we don't know how to help them. We have all been shocked at the apparent increase in child abuse in the last decade or so. I'm not so sure how much of the increase is real and how much just more sensitivity to it. But what have we done about it? Not, for the most part, tried to get at the roots of the problems that threaten family life, that do lead to abuse–factors in our culture. In our living patterns, in our child-rearing practices–despite a few moves in this direction. No, for the most part we have enacted investigatory and punitive laws. We have tried to rescue these children despite the fact that the rescue fantasy is just that–a fantasy. And then we have written the family off. In the name of loving children we have isolated them from their natural milieu, from the only true roots that they have. Talk to an abused child, and you will find that in most cases what he or she wants is not to be rescued from his family but to work out some way in which he can safely return to them. Talk to some so-called abusive parents, and you will find among them concerned and loving people.

It is true that some children need to be away from home for a period of time, sometimes as much for the parent's sake as for their own. Children are not all innocent beings. Sometimes they are a major part of the problem. One of the factors in child abuse is too many children in too little space for too much of the day. Our relationships have become abrasive because they have been too much caught up in the complications of modern life, even the struggle for existence. But it is all too often the family's problem and not the child's and quite certainly not ours. They are the ones who need help and we don't help them or the child by taking over their problems for them. Nor do we help if, as so many child-advocates do, we see the parents as having failed, having lost their rights to be parents, if instead of trying to help with the family's problems, all we do is to break it up. Some families may need to break up so that a new one may grow in its place. But this is an awful and, one might hope, a responsible decision in which parents and child need both to be involved, not something to be accomplished by a well-meaning would-be substitute parent who has assumed the right to make decisions for the child and treats the parents as of no account or importance. This is true even for a judge. Family roots are deep, and in many cases it is to them that the child will return when we have finished with him.

That is why the words "child-centered" have to me a dangerous ring. They are, of course, better than being "institution-centered" or "result-centered" or "public-relation centered," and they were perhaps a necessary stage in the development of a children's agency. They do mean individualizing children, not treating them as a mob or a mass. But to be child-centered is not enough, either, I would like to say, pragmatically or morally. The famous Bellefaire study showed pragmatically what we had long known, and what is really just common sense, that changes in a child's behavior learned in a treatment center were all too easily undone if the agency had tried to treat the child alone, apart from what was happening in his family group. Many a child in placement cannot even begin to work on his own problems until he knows where he stands with his family, something that may take months of concentrated work. Many a child cannot accept substitute parental care, even for a temporary period, until his conflict over his own family has been resolved, which means work with his family about their intentions as well as work with the child, and is, incidentally, one of the reasons why some children move from one foster home to another again and again and again. Many a child still grows up rootless and with little capacity to love and be loved because he was rescued from parents who then were given no meaningful help. There is even some evidence that the well-intentioned movement to find permanency for children whose own families have been allowed to die on the vine through placing them for adoption is running into some difficulty when the child becomes adolescent. Too often that means that the child has not, in his inner self, given his own family up.

But the moral questions are, I think, just as important. They have to do with our whole attitude to people. There are two questions I'd like to ask, and the first is why, in our society, we are so ready to help children and to ignore their parents? Is it because we believe that children can change, and their parents cannot? I don't think so. We seem to be willing to work with alcoholics or criminals, neither very promising clients, and yet, as Maas and Engler pointed out some years ago, most parents whose children are in placement are left to a "self-healing process." We ignore them, or discourage them. No, I think the problem arises from our protective and sentimental instincts, and I would like to say a bit about each. To be protective of someone may be necessary in extremes–there are certain things which should not happen to anyone–and children are, through their immaturity, particularly vulnerable. But protectiveness as an attitude towards others means that deep down one doesn't value the other person. He cannot act for himself. You have to act for him. And children are much more able to face the truth and do something about it than the protective person believes. For every child I have seen hurt by having to face up to things and deal with the problems of his family, I have seen hundreds who were harmed by some well-intentioned protector who wanted to shield him from unhappiness. I am reminded time and again of the girl who became so disturbed after the mother's visits that the Home decided to protect her from them. She turned on the caseworker with the words, "What you don't understand is that this is something I need to be disturbed about."

The same sort of thing is true about sentimentality. It is easy to be sentimental about children, and as a result indignant with anyone we feel to have let them down, but sentimentality is a very self-centered emotion. It is using another person not for his true worth or importance but for your own self-indulgence. It does violence to the other person's integrity, besides being a very poor foundation for action. It is, I think, rather a major sin.

And secondly, since this audience is largely composed of churchmen, I would like to ask what is the proper role of the church when faced with the problems of family life? Is it to be the family, the one who takes over the parental role; or should it be more the extended family, the one who helps, who provides a back-up, who shares but does not presume to take over? Does it care for people or care about them? To care for others, to take over their problems is, I think, a great temptation to pride. It argues that one knows best. It denigrates the person from whom one takes over. The church, in my opinion, has a most vital and important role to play as the extended family. I wish it would play it more often and sometimes with greater charity. But it can and does sometimes rise to the occasion and I have seen it do so beautifully in my own life. Another factor closely related to child abuse, since we have opened that can of worms, is the very lack of someone to share the burden, to relieve one in times of stress; and in this mobile and discontinuous society of ours, the church is perhaps the only institution that can play this role. It does not take over or substitute its wisdom for that of the people it tries to help. That way lies Pride; and Pride, or Superbia, was long ago held by the Church to be the first and the mother of all the Deadly Sins.

It may be unnecessary for me to say this to you. You may already be convinced; and if you know this home you probably are. A good home is truly family-centered, even when it has chosen, among the alternatives open to a Children's Home, the perhaps unenviable task of working with children whose growth has been abnormal, who are, in our somewhat presumptuous vocabulary, disturbed. It spends a great deal of time and effort on and with each individual child. In that sense it is child–centered. Sometimes it may have to insist that the child bear the burden of change, which is unfair (and I hope it says so) but inevitable. It has much better access to the child than to the family and it has the child in its power. But, unless I read it wrong, it never assumes that these are its children. It sees them always as part of a family group. It is concerned, not only that the child shall recover; but that his family should also become the kind of family in which the child can continue to grow, not only for his sake, but for theirs. It is, and I hope that it always will be, family-centered.

Yes, I think there is a real difference in being child-centered and family-centered. To be child-centered is not enough. When, some time ago I was presented with an award that named me a friend of children, undeservably, perhaps, I made the point that one can't really be a friend of children unless one is a friend of adults, too. And I think that in our Children's Homes, and perhaps in social work as a whole, we are just beginning to see that it must be so. We are turning away, slowly, it is true, from taking over people's lives, from passing judgment on them or labeling them as sick or incapable, and entering into partnership with them. We are becoming partners with them rather than those who find out what is wrong and put it right. And I think that there we are discovering something. Many of the people that we have labeled sick or incapable, even parents who have neglected or abused their child, are not so much sick as caught up in pressures that are too much for them to bear; or, if they are sick, they still have a well component which we can help them hold onto. One of the questions we have so often not asked in the past of parents of a disturbed, neglected or abused child, is "Given what has happened, what do you want to do now?" The past is the past. We cannot judge it. We did not walk in your shoes or face the problems that you faced. But life must go on. This is still your child. You are still a family or can be if you want to be. What can you do to help at this time, and how can we help you with it? And, where the question is being asked, sincerely and with a desire to help, there have been some quite surprising results.

Larry Brendtro, the President of the National Association of Homes for Children, said in a speech at Austin recently that the biggest change ahead for Children's Homes was to stop being substitute parents and learn to be supplementary ones–the extended family for those parents and children for whom this world has become, as I think it has, too stressful and complicated for many people to cope with. Another friend of mine, Ed Lowenstein, believes that within a few years the vast majority of people will need help–not just the sick, the oppressed, the failures–but people like you and me who find themselves confronted with so complicated a world, so many conflicting values and so many roles to play for which we are unprepared that we almost literally do not know which way to turn. In fact he says that such help will be routine, necessary and universal. And probably the most complicated, the most vulnerable and the most rapidly changing of all social institutions is the American family. It is, unfortunately, also the most violent. If indeed the whole concept of family is to survive in our society, it needs all the help that we can give it.

We in the church care about families–or, at least we say we do. We are, or should be, family-centered. We cannot allow our sentimentality, our partisanship, far less our desire to take over, our judgementalism, our righteous or unrighteous indignation, our protectiveness, to aid in the dissolution of something we believe in. What we need is not a Year of the Child but a Year of the Family. When that comes along I'll say, "Yes, God, yes."

REFERENCES

Melvin E. Allerhand, Ruth E. Weber and Marie Haug. *Adaptation and Adaptability: The Bellefaire Follow-Up Study* (New York 1966).
Henry Maas and Richard Engler. *Children in Need of Parents* (New York 1959).
Edward R. Lowenstein. "Social Work in a Post-Industrial Society," *Social Work* 18, 6 (Nov. 1973) 47.

BIOGRAPHICAL NOTE

Dr. Keith-Lucas was a social worker for more than fifty years as a practitioner, administrator, educator, and prolific writer. His particular interests were in the group care of children, the history and philosophy of social work, and the integration of religious faith and social work practice. He published more than 20 books and monographs, in addition to more than 150 professional articles or chapters in books. He was a consultant to more than 100 children's homes. He "retired" officially from the University of North Carolina School of Social Work as Alumni Distinguished Professor but continued to remain active as a scholar, consultant and Editor of the Book Review Section of this journal until his death in 1995. Children remember him chiefly as a teller of Uncle Remus stories.

"On Runaway"

Several times during the year
he made an appointment
saying he wanted to see me.
but he didn't show
for he was a runaway kid

Or maybe he came occasionally
staying for five restless minutes
before leaving to run away again
instead of a year in residence
his had been a runaway year.

Once more his name was in the book
put there at his request
when he came, restlessly
I asked if he would like to walk
so we went on walkaway
together, around the grounds

Down the lane by the dumpster
across the swinging bridge
across the edge of the reedy swamp
over to the big bass pond
and back along the creek
pushing through the willow clumps

He was the trusted guide, out front
knowing every step of the way
holding back the branches
to keep them from slapping
the face of the one who followed

[Haworth co-indexing entry note]: "On Runaway." Powers, Douglas. Co-published simultaneously in *Residential Treatment for Children & Youth* (The Haworth Press, Inc.) Vol. 17, No. 3, 2000, pp. 11-12; and: *Family-Centered Services in Residential Treatment: New Approaches for Group Care* (ed: John Y. Powell) The Haworth Press, Inc., 2000, pp. 11-12. Single or multiple copies of this article are available for a fee from The Haworth Document Delivery Service [1-800-342-9678, 9:00 a.m. - 5:00 p.m. (EST). E-mail address: getinfo@haworthpressinc.com].

He identified the wild flowers
pointed where the ground was firm
described the habits of a praying mantis
discovered fingerlings fanning
in a hidden pool of the creek
pointed to places where doves nested

This is a place I come to
sometimes when I run away
it's a good place to think
and to cool off when you're mad
he confided while holding limbs
that were about to spring

Coming back across the bridge
he suggested we play Racing Sticks
so we each threw a small stick
into the creek above the bridge
and when they came in view downstream
they were floating side by side
as if held together by unseen force

Hey, we both won, he said, with a smile
that contained a here and now expression
and not a far away runaway look

We parted at the turn off to his cottage
where he stopped and hesitated a moment
then said, I think I'll put my name
down in your book for the other days
that you're here, if its all right.
it was all right, and he was there
runaways decreased from many to rare.

Douglas Powers, MD

Reinventing Residential Childcare:
An Agenda for Research and Practice

James K. Whittaker, PhD

SUMMARY. Until recently, "residential childcare" in North America was, for a variety of reasons, more likely to be seen as part of the "problem" as opposed to the "solution" for most child and family problems. Thus, the development of residential care theory, innovative practices and research all languished as the spotlight of interest focused on such "newer" service developments as "intensive family preservation services," "treatment foster care," and "wrap-around services." As Corbillon (1993) notes, the neglect, in particular, of an integrated set of research priorities for residential childcare is a problem for at least some European countries (France) as well. Recently, the spectre of children orphaned by AIDS, the somewhat disappointing research results from family based service initiatives and the challenges posed by children and youth who present multiple problems including serious emotional disturbance, substance abuse, and a history of violence have worked to stimulate a renewed interest in residential care and treatment. This presentation will briefly review the "developmental history" of residential care in a North American context and identify several chal-

Originally delivered as a plenary presentation for the 6th Congress of the European Scientific Society for Residential and Foster Care for Children and Adolescents [EUSARF], 23-26 September, 1998, University of Paris-X Nanterre. Earlier versions of portions of the paper were presented at the Duke Symposium on group care, East Carolina University, School of Social Work, April 10-11, 1997 and a working conference of the New York City Aids Orphan Project: *Planning & Placement: Expanding the Options for Orphans of the HIV Epidemic*, Fund for the City of New York, October 17-18, 1996.

Dr. James K. Whittaker, Professor of Social Work, may be written at the University of Washington, Seattle, WA 98195.

13

lenges for research in the areas of residential program design and definition, assessment and intake, and outcomes and community aftercare. The article concludes with a series of specific recommendations for residential childcare innovation, theory development, and research prioritization. *[Article copies available for a fee from The Haworth Document Delivery Service: 1-800-342-9678. E-mail address: getinfo@haworthpressinc.com <Website: http://www.haworthpressinc.com>]*

KEYWORDS. Reinventing residential care, residential childcare, group childcare, innovations in residential childcare

The author wishes to express sincere thanks to the following individual members of EUSARF for the invitation to present to the EUSARF Congress as well as for their many contributions to theory and research in residential youth care: Dr. Michael Corbillon, of Universite Paris Ys., Nanterre, the Scientific Committee president and Congress chairman; Prof. Paul Durning also of the Universite Paris X, Nanterre; Prof. Walter Hellinckx, of Leuven University, Belgium, the current president of EUSARF; and Professor J. D. van der Ploeg, Dr. E. Scholte, Dr. Erik Knorth, and Dr. M. Smit, all of Leiden University, The Netherlands.

I am honored to participate in what looks like a veritable "feast of ideas" on better ways of serving children and their families. In particular, I look forward to a lively discussion on a long neglected topic in child welfare: residential care and treatment.

As a North American scholar, I am acutely aware of the cultural bias and limitations that I bring in my perspectives on child and family practice and research. I will speak from what I know best and leave it to each of you–the delegates–to decide what is relevant for the European scene. I do know enough to realize that the "Euro" label contains within it much diversity-cultural, political, regional, religious, national and ethnic–which must be attended to in any comprehensive assessment of residential and foster care.

I commend EUSARF for choosing substitute care, in particular, residential care as the primary focus for this Congress. I am pained to say that I know of no such parallel meetings in North America, save for those perennial discussions which define residential care as more a problem than a solution.

In it simplest form, my message to you is: North American group care needs your help. Those few of us who are committed to the notion of a renewed residential care sector desperately need the considerable European practice, research, and policy expertise that is represented in this room. My personal hope is that this EUSARF Congress will serve as the catalyst for a broad ranging North American discussion of substitute care: a discussion that is long overdue.

Ironically, one of the very few recent serious considerations of residential care which I am aware was stimulated by the spectre of AIDS, that terrifying and insidious disease that has had more to do with altering the face of every "system" (from drug approval, to health and social services) with which it has come in contact than any reform initiative in my memory. In this instance, the growing numbers of children orphaned by AIDS in New York City and surrounding areas is causing re-examination of an old and unresolved issue: the care and nurture of dependent children when "family" (at least, "family" in the conventional sense) is not an option. I was recently privileged to work with a small and diverse group consisting of social historians, child welfare experts, AIDS services providers and adults who had spent a significant part of their formative years in substitute care. The report of the NY AIDS Orphan Project is now available (Levine, Brandt, & Whittaker, 1998) and I will return to those sections most relevant to our discussions at a later point.

In my brief time with you this morning, I would like to address three interrelated topics pertaining to residential, or group childcare:

1. To begin, I will offer a brief summary of what I take to be current "conventional wisdom" with respect to residential care in North America and address some of the attendant causes and consequences of this thinking.
2. Next, I will offer a very brief "sketch" of demographics, service trends, and outcome research in residential childcare, and
3. Finally, I will identify three domains of critical problem solving for residential group care and touch briefly on each:

   - The first has to do with the "definition and purpose" of residential care in an overall continuum of child and family service.
   - Next, "intake" and what youth are best served by residential placement, and

- Third, "outcome" indicators: What are reasonable outcomes for the multiple forms of residential care and treatment that presently exist?

I will conclude with several brief recommendations for innovations in residential care practice and research which, I believe, will further our understanding of each of these three domains.

I approach this international Congress feeling "deep" in some subject areas (such as contemporary residential care practice in the U.S.), while facing a very "steep learning curve" in others (such as the cultural/political histories that have shaped residential care provision in the variety of European states represented here). I suspect I am not alone.

Fortunately, Dr. Corbillon and the Congress planning committee have provided us with the opportunity to view residential care and fostering through many different lenses: cross national and cross cultural, as well from the perspectives of policy, evaluative research, and actual practice. Hopefully, as we struggle to comprehend some of the "parts," the "whole" (i.e., the place and purpose of residential care and fostering in contemporary child and family services) will become more clear.

At the outset, I must share with you *three interconnected experiences in my own lifecourse* and the influence these have had on the development of my perspectives on child and family services including residential care:

1. I began my career in residential childcare as a direct care worker in a small residential treatment center in New England, the Walker Home for Children, in the early 1960s while still a student at university. Our training manual for staff lives on as the volume *The Other 23 Hours* (Trieschman, Whittaker, & Brendtro, 1969), and reflects our best thinking at the time on how one goes about organizing a "therapeutic milieu." Later, at a university affiliated summer training camp for troubled children, The University of Michigan Fresh Air Camp, whose founders included Fritz Redl and David Wineman, I learned at first hand the meaning of the term: "L'ennfant Aggressif."

These "early experiences" left an indelible imprint: No matter how grand our theoretical models of treatment, or how elegant our research designs for measuring outcomes, the ultimate test of "success" in residential care depends entirely on the quality and effectiveness of the relationship of those care staff who are in daily, direct, intimate, face-to-face contact with troubled children and youth.

2. For the past 28 years, my wife and I have struggled to understand the meaning of what it is to be the parents of a "special needs" child (now a young adult):

- To realize, first, that while we had both worked with disturbed children, nothing in our professional clinical training or education prepared us adequately for what it was like to be parents of a child who, in some significant ways, was profoundly different from other children.
- Secondly, to experience the enormous power differential that exists between "professionals" and "parents" and how even helpful professional interventions can add to what Bernheim (1982) calls "family burden."
- Thirdly, to reflect on our journey of parenthood, help has come in some unusual ways and from some unlikely places. *My attitudes towards parents, peers, indeed towards "lay helping" of all kinds has been profoundly altered by my personal parental experience which is still unfolding. As we talk in this Congress about the "ingredients" of helpful interventions, we would do well to be mindful of the observation of Jean Vanier that help need not be "extraordinary" or "heroic," but consists primarily of doing "ordinary things with tenderness."*

3. Lastly, in my continuing work as a practice researcher and consultant in child and family services, I am continually made aware that the development of innovative practice models whether in residential care or other service domains represents only half of the task. The other, far more challenging work involves the creation and maintenance of what I'll call the "organizational infra-structure" of effective practice. This includes, but is not limited to:

- supervision, staff training and the development of coherent practice protocols,
- well-designed program evaluation including specification of socially significant outcomes, and development of processes

and procedures for the continuous monitoring and quality improvement of practices.
- Political advocacy including development of reliable funding and promotion of good community relations.

For the last dozen or so years, I have joined with a team of national research consultants in working with a large establishment in our middle west that serves several thousand delinquent youth and their families in a wide variety of service programs [Boysville of Michigan]. We are committed to building a model of research based youth service. *This experience provides me with abundant humility in realizing how difficult it is to change existing systems, how challenging it is to translate "research" into terms that have practical meaning and how much all of our service improvement efforts rise or fall on the tide of changing political whim or unforeseen events.*

Now, we return to our main topic, residential care. *Question: What is the "conventional wisdom" about residential care in the North America?* Answer: Now, it is more typically seen as a service one uses as a last resort. Often, residential care is viewed more as part of the problem, rather than as part of the solution.

This is so for a variety of reasons:

1. *Lack of diagnostic indicators.* The identification of a scientifically based diagnostic criteria for residential placement continues to elude us.
2. *A presumed preference within some service systems for placement without first attempting some less radical community and family based interventions.*
3. *A presumption of "intrusiveness" and concerns about attachment for children placed.*
4. *Fear of abuse and neglect within residential settings.*
5. *Questionable effectiveness of residential treatment.*
6. *A lack of consensus on critical intervention components.*
7. *A lack of residential treatment theory development, particularly in recent years.*
8. *Cost of care.*
9. *A continuing familial bias in service selection.*

Since at the least the first decade of this century, there exists a presumption that residential care if used at all ought to be seen as a "last resort" (i.e., when all other options are exhausted).

This is particularly so when child dependency is the primary issue. Preference should go to foster family care, adoption, guardianship or other alternatives. On this last point, there has been near unanimity over the course of my career: Children who are purely "dependent/neglected" should not be served in group care settings.

In fact, the most single stable trend line in child welfare over the last 75+ years is the shifting ratio of children in foster family vs. residential care as a proportion of the total number of children in out-of-home care. So for example, as Kadushin (1980) notes from approximately the early 1930s to the mid 1970s, the percentage of children in residential care declined from 57% to 15%, while the percentage in family foster care increased from 43% to 85% for the total population of children served in out-of-home care. Thus, despite an increase in the rate of placement and in the ratio of children out-of-home to those served in-home, the proportions of children in residential vs. foster family care options have remained relatively constant.

With a few regional exceptions (for example, the southeastern United States), the following description of group care offered by turn of the century reformer, Hastings Hart, that "institutional life is contrary to child nature" seems to have held sway in public policy and practice. Then, late in 1994 the "new orphan" issue burst on the American scene in early December, just in time to make a catchy story for Christmas!

First, a conservative Republican landslide in our federal congress highlighted a policy agenda termed "The Contract with America" which contained within it a provision to return to the orphanage model as a safe haven for some children abused and neglected by their parental caretakers. The "debate" carried out in mainstream print and electronic media included the Speaker of the House (Newt Gingrich) urging the First Lady (Hillary Clinton) to rent the 1940s movie *Boy's Town* presumably to glean some lessons for family policy from Spencer Tracy and Mickey Rooney! (Not widely reported at the time was the comment of one of these new found experts on family–Mickey Rooney–to the effect that being married 8 times made for some confusion at Christmas and other major holidays, in that one was never quite sure where one should be!)

This was set in the context of a growing backlash against "family preservation": a topic widely discussed in the last two EUSARF Congresses and thought of in North America as services designed to prevent the *unnecessary* placement of children into care while continuing to provide for their safety. People like Patrick Murphy, Children's Advocate in Cook County (Chicago), and Richard Gelles, leading family violence researcher, urged serious consideration of alternative out-of-home care settings for certain children for whom family was neither a safe nor viable long term option. In point of fact, little happened to change conventional wisdom.

Government policy since then has been even more supportive of family based alternatives (e.g., adoption incentives) for children for whom there is little hope of return to parents of origin. At the level of individual states, "family group conferencing" originating in New Zealand has replaced intensive family preservation service as the "cutting edge" of practice innovation (Connolly & McKenzie, 1999). Serious discussions of group care options for long term care occur only at the margins of policy and practice debate. No one seriously entertains the option of return to the "orphanage" model with all of its negative connotations. What is most significant to me is that the issue came up at all: perhaps, providing a brief glimpse of a well-masked anxiety over our infatuation with family based service delivery.

OVERVIEW OF CONTEMPORARY RESIDENTIAL CARE IN THE U.S.

The previously mentioned lack of interest in residential care is reflected in administrative data gathering as well. Despite several exciting initiatives in federal and state data gathering in children's services (e.g., U.S. DHHS, 1997), it is still difficult to compile an up-to-date and accurate picture of group care.

I will offer only a few general observations here. Please see some of the source documents listed in the references for more. From our latest census and other sources, we do know the following:

1. While the numbers of children residing in substitute care are small in proportion to the total child population (less than 1%), they are increasingly troubled and present multiple problems at intake.

2. Anywhere between 15% and 30% of the out of home care population resides in residential as opposed to foster family care.
3. We have more residential facilities, albeit with smaller sized living units.
4. Lengths of stay are shorter and children are, on average, older at intake.
5. In certain sectors, we are seeing more proprietary agencies (e.g., children's psychiatric facilities) and more specialized facilities (e.g., those serving youth with substance abuse problems, and problems related to sexual offending).
6. Among residential centers (many of which are voluntary), we are seeing more mergers, more closures and less stability with respect to funding.
7. There is a growing emphasis on specification of standardized child and family outcomes and, not surprisingly, more emphasis on specification of treatment and care protocols. In large measure this influence is positive, though in certain types of residential facilities, some have used the term "medicalization" to describe what is happening to residential programs as they strive to meet criteria for psychiatric reimbursement.

At the level of actual residential practice, the clinical equivalent of the "holy wars" (e.g., between psychoanalytic, psycho-educational, behavioral and positive peer culture approaches) has receded into the background. There is instead a much more eclectic, nondogmatic, perhaps atomistic approach to practice, as programs struggle to meet the highly prescriptive outcome and procedural requirements of their contracts. The resultant aggregation of program components–each targeted to a particular youth problem–often yields a structure that, in my judgment, lacks coherence as a total milieu. I am reminded here of the observation of one of my favorite historians of science, Steven Jay Gould of Harvard, who describes an exclusive reliance on inductive processes in science as akin to constructing a building, brick-by-brick, without a blueprint. Much of current residential care in the States is being built "brick-by-brick" without a blueprint. Let us turn now to the question of outcome research and what is "known" about residential care. I will offer only the briefest overview here from an American context. [Please note as well the excellent research reviews referenced in the handout including the EUSARF volume *Innovations in Resi-*

dential Child Care (Hellinckx, Broekaert, Vanden Berge, & Colton, 1991) and the excellent U.K. review authored by Roger Bullock, Michael Little and Spencer Millham for the Dartington group (1993).] Perhaps, a good place to begin from a U.S. perspective is with the recent report of our Government Accounting Office (U.S. GAO, 1994), the office charged with answering questions posed by members of congress on a wide variety of policy related topics. Typically their reports involve synthesis of existing research as well as conducting original studies. Here is a statement from their executive summary:

> Not enough is known about residential care programs to provide a clear picture of which kinds of treatment approaches work best or about the effectiveness of the treatment over the long term. Further, no consensus exists on which youths are best served by residential care . . . or how residential care should be combined with community based care to best serve at risk youths over time. (p. 4)

This report identifies eleven characteristics which appear to be related to success: (1) developing individual treatment plans, (2) participation of a caring adult, (3) self-esteem building, (4) planning for post-program living, (5) teaching social, coping and living skills, (6) coordination of services, (7) involving the family, (8) positive peer influence, (9) enforcing a strict code of discipline, (10) post-program support, and (11) providing a family-like atmosphere.

While these are socially significant as indicators of presumed "best practices," not all share the same degree of empirical validation. Among those that do appear to be supported by outcome studies are: (1) involving a parent or other concerned adult in the client's care, and (2) planning adequate supports for the youth's return to the community after completing the program. Support for these findings are noted in several recent reviews of residential care research (Curry, 1993; Whittaker & Pfeiffer, 1994) and underscore the importance of contact and involvement with family during the placement period and, more generally, on the importance of supports in the post-discharge environment. For example, a follow-up study, by Dr. Kathleen Wells (Wells, Wyatt, & Hobfoll, 1991), formerly research director at Bellefaire–a well known residential treatment center in Cleveland, Ohio–repeats the classic follow-up research conducted in that same agency in the 1960s (Allerhand, Weber, & Haug, 1966). Dr. Wells concludes as follows:

> A failure to respond in some way to the conditions in the environments in which youths were discharged may well undo the hard won gains youths make in treatment. . . . We need . . . the reconceptualization of residential treatment as a family support system and to identify the potential stressors and stability of the environments to which youth are returned. (1991, p. 214)

As Curry notes (1993), in an insightful review paper, we are learning more about the various domains of social support and their relationship to adaptive outcomes for youth:

> Results (of the Wells et al. study, 1991) showed that measures of adaptation were positively intercorrelated, but measures of social support were not. Thus, while a youngster tending to function well in one area was likely to function well in others, sources of support were not necessarily correlated. Support from family members was most strongly related to psychological adaptation. (p. 13)

Curry concludes by affirming the importance of increasing family support in the post-discharge period and suggests that alternative sources of support may not fully compensate for lack of family support.

So what can be said, at this point from the existing research base with respect to residential care? A recent review suggests three things:

1. Regardless of a youth's status at discharge, the quality of supports available in the post-discharge environment appears to be associated with subsequent community adjustment.
2. Continuing contact and involvement with family appears to be positively correlated with post-placement success.
3. Youths with supportive community networks are more likely to maintain their treatment gains than those who lack such supports. (Pecora, Whittaker, & Maluccio, 1992, p. 421)

I am hopeful because a number of imaginative residential practitioners and innovative agencies have created some interesting options in the last several years for both engaging families more fully while providing support for youth. A soon to be published paper by the Child Welfare League of America documents these efforts for those who might be interested in further detail (Whittaker, in press).

As residential programs move forward to adopt and adapt many of the family focused practice innovations from these and related projects, it is critical that these be accompanied by rigorous evaluations to insure their relationship to the ultimate outcomes of interest: community adjustment and integration for youths returning from care (Whittaker & Savas, 1999). Researchers and practitioners alike will face several critical challenges in providing empirical validation for family-agency partnerships. These include, but are not limited to:

1. *Developing Protocols for Family Practice.* At present, no clear consensus exists in the field with respect to the locus of family engagement (in-home, agency based, community based); the focus of the engagement (family treatment, counseling, education); the format (telephone contact vs. face to face, group vs. individual), the knowledge and skills required of the family worker; or the sequencing of the intervention. For example, are there advantages/disadvantages to "front-loading" or "back-loading" family involvement for youth in care? The training capacity for enhanced family work must also be further specified and empirically validated if the field is to move beyond simply enumerating the "values and principles" of a family focused approach (Ainsworth, Maluccio, & Small, 1996).

2. *Developing Rapid Assessment/Brief Intervention Models for Family Work.* The increasing influence of managed care with its emphasis on shorter term residential programming highlights the need for adaptation of assessment and intervention protocols to meet the shorter time frames. Such time pressures underscore the point made by many commentators on the importance of constructing a seamless path of family involvement beginning with pre-placement and extending through placement into aftercare activity (Jenson & Whittaker, 1989).

3. *Developing Family Work that is Effective with Special Populations and Which Reflects Appropriate Cultural and Ethnic Variation.* The previously cited report on children orphaned by AIDS highlighted special considerations for such children in out-of-home placements (Levine, Brandt, & Whittaker, 1998).

Similarly, family engagement strategies for youths who present dual diagnoses and or who are involved (or whose families are involved) in recovery may require customization of family work to fit their particular needs. Finally, as the previously cited CWLA report (Braziel, 1996) notes, "families" represent a spectrum of cultural and ethnic diversity and effective work with them will require a solid grounding in cultural competence as well as family practice technique (cited in Leigh, 1998).

4. *Documenting the Link Between Family Support Intervention and Youth Outcomes.* While the existing corpus of residential outcome research leads us ineluctably to work on improving agency-family partnerships, it remains to be documented how increasing familial support actually improves and enhances youth outcomes. With the growing trend towards outcome based contracting, it is critical that we increase our understanding of the mechanisms by which a supportive (and well supported) family serves to buffer the adverse effects of the otherwise stark community environments to which youth must all too often return following residential placement.

I believe our greatest challenge in these and in all other areas of residential research is that we take care to match theory based and well crafted and innovative residential practice with the appropriate choice of our increasingly diverse evaluative research methods. Otherwise, we run the risk of subjecting what is essentially the "best of the past" (in residential practice) to research analysis characterized by increasing rigor and sophistication.

Let me turn now to the final section of my paper.

THREE CRITICAL AREAS OF PROBLEM SOLVING FOR RESIDENTIAL CARE

Out-of-home placement for children in general and residential childcare specifically presents us with a series of interrelated problems:

Problems of Definition

- What precisely do we mean by the variety of forms of service that make up the spectrum of out-of-home care: group homes; intensive residential treatment; therapeutic foster care?

- What are the critical elements in and defining characteristics of each?
- How do we balance and integrate care and treatment needs of children? What implications do each raise specific to group residential care settings?

I reiterate here my plea for more focused work on theoretical model development in residential care. I believe there is some danger that as we move from "service" centered planning to "child/family" centered planning, we will lose a needed focus on residential care as a total intervention. In my judgment, both types of planning are needed if we are truly to understand the power of the residential milieu and then use it in creative ways to meet specific clinical and developmental needs of individual children and their families.

Problems of Intake

- For what types of child behavior problems is residential care or other forms of placement the "treatment of choice" as opposed to "the last resort?"
- What are the "offsets" to some of the presumed negatives associated with placement (e.g., separation from family/community/culture):–*intensity* of the treatment provided?–the *physical safety* of the child? *protection* for the community?

Residential care is an expensive, complex, and radical intervention. It should be used judiciously and where it can achieve the most good. To achieve this will require some critical rethinking of conventional wisdom. For example, for an individual youth whose life trajectory is headed towards adult incarceration, maybe, as Mary Beth Curtis of Boy's Town notes, the "least restrictive environment" is the one in which most growth (academic, social, physical) can occur for the immediate future and/or where "safe passage" may be provided.

Problems of Outcome

- What span of indicators signal "success" in residential care?
- At what time points should they be measured and where?
- Should there be a "statute of limitations" on residential outcomes?

Discussion of "outcomes" is proceeding at a very fast pace in the U.S. right now, largely as a result of fascination with "managed care." In the residential arena, while there have been some benefits that derive solely from the outcomes discussion (a focus on realistic and well specified goal setting, for example), it is clear that *any* discussion of outcomes must be linked to a discussion of intake and program design issues as well. Otherwise, some residential establishments may find themselves being held accountable for child and family outcomes in areas where they are service-deficient, or for promising "results" in cases where they have inadequately assessed both risk and acuity.

RECOMMENDATIONS

I wish to end with a few specific prescriptions for residential care in the U.S. The remedies are partial and to a certain degree idiosyncratic and I have no illusion that they constitute a panacea. I believe collectively they will increase the likelihood of finding answers to many of the questions I have posed regarding residential care.

First and foremost, I believe we need to design a new service continuum that softens the differences and blurs the boundaries between in-home and out-of-home options such as shared care, respite care, and partial placements. Kinship care may be a step in that direction.

Some other things that would be helpful include:

- Re-doubling our efforts at parent involvement.
- Expanding residential respite options.
- Developing more creative short term residential treatment.
- Focusing on child well being and family functioning as outcome measures.
- Studying honestly the limits as well as the potential of family centered service delivery.
- Developing models of whole family care, for example, by combining respite with holiday time and skill building for families.
- Working to personalize residential care settings and reinforce primary caregivers.
- Examining the potential for the co-location of services: e.g., family support and residential care.
- Seeking partners and being able to locate our residential programs in an overall service network.

- Conduct longitudinal research to study developmental outcomes for youth in shared care and those temporarily placed.
- Re-designing some group care settings for permanent living and re-examining communal alternatives (e.g., Israeli cluster foster care).

The previously cited New York City AIDS Orphan Project (Levine et al., 1998) reached the tentative conclusion that group residential care ought to be at least *one* option open to children made orphans by the disease. Such group care settings, it was argued, ought to meet five basic criteria:

1. Continuity of developmentally appropriate caregiving with stable caregivers.
2. Maintaining stability of sibling groups.
3. Providing a structured and predictable environment.
4. Maintenance of meaningful connections with "family."
5. Continuity with community and culture.

CONCLUSION

I am pessimistic about achieving even a few of these modest changes in my country absent a more focused and thoughtful discussion on substitute care as a whole. My strong sense is that we need to bring the worlds of policy, research and practice in residential and foster care into much closer proximity so that we can assess what the challenges and strengths are in each domain and then chart a course of action for renewal. We sorely need European perspectives on these issues to broaden and stimulate our limited and parochial discussions in the states. Again, I hope that EUSARF can play a key role in extending the spirit and substance of this Congress to a wider audience and I am committed to doing whatever I can to make this happen.

REFERENCES

Ainsworth, F., Maluccio, A.N., & Small, R.W. (1996). A framework for family-centered group care practice: Guiding principles and practice applications. In D.J. Braziel (Ed.), *Family-focused practice in out-of-home care* (pp. 35-45). Washington, DC: Child Welfare League of America.

Allerhand, M.E., Weber, G., & Haug, M. (1966). *Adaptation and adaptability: The Bellefaire follow up study.* New York: Child Welfare League of America.

Bernheim, K. (1982). Supportive family counseling. *Schizophrenic Bulletin, 8*, 634-641.

Bullock, R., Little, M., & Milham, S. (1993). *Residential care of children: A review of the research.* London: HMSO.

Braziel, D.J. (Ed.). (1996). *Family-focused practice in out-of-home care.* Washington, DC: Child Welfare League of America.

Connolly, M., & McKenzie, M. (1999). *Effective participatory practice: Family group conferencing in child protection.* New York: Aldine de Gruyter.

Curry, J. (1991). Outcome research on residential treatment: Implications and suggested directions. *American Journal of Orthopsychiatry, 61*, 348-358.

Hellinckx, W., Broekaert, E., Vanden Berge, A., & Colton, M. (Eds.). (1991). *Innovations in residential care.* Acco Leuven, Netherlands: Amersfoort.

Jenson, J., & Whittaker, J. K. (1987). Parental involvement in children's residential treatment: From pre-placement to aftercare. *Children and Youth Services Review,* 9(2), 81-100.

Kadushin, A. (1980). *Child welfare services* (3rd ed.). New York: Macmillan.

Leigh, J.W. (1998). *Communicating for cultural competence.* New York: Allyn & Bacon.

Levine, C.I., Brandt, A., & Whittaker, J.K. (1998). *Staying together, living apart: New perspectives on youth group living from the AIDS epidemic* (from Planning and Placement Project). (Available from Carol Levine, The United Hospital Fund, 23rd Floor, 350 Fifth Avenue, New York, NY 10118, U.S.A.)

Pecora, P.J., Whittaker, J.K., & Maluccio, A.N. (1992). *The child welfare challenge. Policy, practice, and research.* New York: Aldine de Gruyter.

Trieschman, A.E., Whittaker, J.K., & Brendtro, L.K. (1969). *The other 23 hours: Child care work with emotional disturbed children in a therapeutic milieu.* New York: Aldine de Gruyter.

U.S. Department of Health and Human Services, Children's Bureau. (1997). *National study of protective, preventive, and reunification services delivered to children and their families.* Washington, DC: U.S. Government Printing Office.

U.S. General Accounting Office. (1994). *Residential care: Some high-risk youth benefit, but more study needed.* (Available from GAO, P.O. Box 6015, Gaithersburg, No 20884-6015, U. S. A.)

Wells, K., Wyatt, E., & Hobfoll, S. (1991). Factors associated with adaptation of youths discharged from residential treatment. *Children and Youth Services Review, 13*, 199-216.

Whittaker, J.K. (in press). Family partnerships in residential child care and treatment: Empirical support/practice challenge. In M. Kluger, G. Alexander, & P. Curtis (Eds.), *What works in child welfare?* Washington, DC: Child Welfare League of America.

Whittaker, J.K., & Pfeiffer, S.I. (1994). Research priorities for residential group child care. *Child Welfare, 73*, 583-601.

Whittaker, J.K., & Savas, S.A. (1999). Community links for troubled youth: A neglected dimension in service planning. In E. Knorth & M. Smit (Eds.), *Handbook on structured residential care* (English version). Leuven-Apeldoorn, Netherlands: Garant.

BIOGRAPHICAL NOTE

Dr. James K. Whittaker is Professor of Social Work at the University of Washington (Seattle). Dr. Whittaker's outstanding and vast contributions to the literature of residential treatment span over thirty years. *The Other 23 Hours* (with Albert E. Trieschman and Larry K. Brendtro, 1969) began as the staff manual of Walker School, where he was then employed. A classic, it continues in print and is available in several languages. His *Caring for Troubled Children* (1979) was recently reprinted in paperback. He continues to challenge readers with his insightful and often prophetic observations. He also serves as a consultant and board member to several residential treatment and group care agencies.

"Migrate"

He looked at the word
Spelled out: M I G R A T E.
Migrate, he sounded,
With a question mark.

Yes. That's right.
Do you know what that means?

It means Johnny Scruggs.

Johnny Scruggs?
I don't understand.

Johnny Scruggs always says,
Every home run he hits,
"Look at me, look at me.
Boy, MIGRATE, MIGRATE."

Douglas Powers, MD

[Haworth co-indexing entry note]: "Migrate." Powers, Douglas. Co-published simultaneously in *Residential Treatment for Children & Youth* (The Haworth Press, Inc.) Vol. 17, No. 3, 2000, p. 31; and: *Family-Centered Services in Residential Treatment: New Approaches for Group Care* (ed: John Y. Powell) The Haworth Press, Inc., 2000, p. 31. Single or multiple copies of this article are available for a fee from The Haworth Document Delivery Service [1-800-342-9678, 9:00 a.m. - 5:00 p.m. (EST). E-mail address: getinfo@haworthpressinc.com].

Family-Centered Practice in Residential Treatment Settings: A Parent's Perspective

Sandra Spencer, BA
John Y. Powell, PhD

Sandra Spencer is a parent of a child with serious emotional disturbances (SED) and also is a family advocate, serving as the Executive Director of WE-CARE (With Every Child and Adult Reaching Excellence), a Greenville, NC, based family support organization. Ms. Spencer travels extensively speaking on behalf of children and families, and she recently testified before the US Congress regarding the urgent need for comprehensive and quality community-based and family-centered children's mental health services. She was interviewed for this article by John Y. Powell.

Interviewer: The readers of *Residential Treatment for Children & Youth* would be interested in having your perspective as a parent. Stephen has been placed in two residential treatment settings: first in a near-by community-based center, and later in an in-patient unit at a university hospital over one hundred miles away.

Ms. Spencer: It is difficult to realize that your son needed to be taken out of your care and placed in a residential home; it was really

Ms. Sandra Spencer, Executive Director, may be written at WE-CARE, Inc., 319-C Saint Andrews Drive, Greenville, NC 27834.

[Haworth co-indexing entry note]: "Family-Centered Practice in Residential Treatment Settings: A Parent's Perspective." Spencer, Sandra and John Y. Powell. Co-published simultaneously in *Residential Treatment for Children & Youth* (The Haworth Press, Inc.) Vol. 17, No. 3, 2000, pp. 33-43; and: *Family-Centered Services in Residential Treatment: New Approaches for Group Care* (ed: John Y. Powell) The Haworth Press, Inc., 2000, pp. 33-43. Single or multiple copies of this article are available for a fee from The Haworth Document Delivery Service [1-800-342-9678, 9:00 a.m. - 5:00 p.m. (EST). E-mail address: getinfo@haworthpressinc.com].

© 2000 by The Haworth Press, Inc. All rights reserved.

hard for me because he was only four-and-a-half years old at the time. And so I thought, "Boy, that is kind of young." The community treatment center had never had a kid under five to be placed there. He was entering kindergarten, but there was no way he could function in a public school. The hardest part of placement in most residential homes is that they have a rule that during the first week or so they don't want visitation because they want the kids to adjust and to get the feel of the place without having the parents in and out.

That did not make sense to me; I pleaded with them because Stephen was so young. But I thought even if he were fifteen I would have had a hard time with that. They did eventually bend the rules a little. I feared that he would feel abandoned . . . taking him somewhere and leaving him, not seeing him for a week. Because I insisted, I did get to visit him a couple of times that first week, but they were short visits. I would do things like go in and read him his bedtime story and then go home, or stop by and eat lunch with him–things like that. And that helped me, and I hope it helped him. The positive for me was that the first residential home was only ten minutes from my house. It is overwhelming for families whose kids are two and three hours away–and sometimes even in a different state. I hear a lot about that–of families who put their kids in residential homes but live so far that they can only visit on weekends or a couple times a month. So, I was fortunate that he wasn't far away. But, on a positive note, I really was glad that he was going to be in a safe environment and there were going to be people who could watch him around the clock, and then they could really assess him 24 hours a day. They would see how he reacted in the school environment and during leisure time: I felt like they could teach me a lot about what was going on with him and how I might handle it.

Interviewer: Did that happen?

Ms. Spencer: That happened some. I found out that families had to continue to go and continue to ask. This wasn't something that just happened. They expected me to come in once a week for what they call "family therapy." So I would go in every Friday afternoon to do family therapy. They would sit around and talk about how Stephen and I could better interact and suggest some things we could do at home. But I wanted to know, in addition to that, was how he was getting along at the group home; how he was getting along with the other kids; if they were seeing the same problems at the group home that I was seeing at home. Because I had been made to feel that Stephen was having all of these difficulties at home because I didn't know the proper discipline techniques, and I didn't have enough structure in my home. I really thought, if that's the case, there must be some environmental thing, and there's nothing wrong with my child. They were really hesitant sometimes about sharing all the information with me. Finally we made up a little behavior report card where they would let me know that "Stephen had these behaviors today, and this is what we had to do." It was validating for me because he was in a treatment group home and he was still having difficulties with his behaviors all during the day: They had a behavior grading system for the kids. They called them "steps," and the first step was "crawling." But I really did not know what the terms stood for . . .

Interviewer: Did anyone tell you at the beginning what they *meant?*

Ms. Spencer: No. When Stephen would come home on the weekends sometimes he would say, "Mom I was 'flying high' today." And I thought, "what's flying high?" Or "I was 'crawling' today." So I had to go and find out. I said to them that if they would teach family members the techniques they were using and how they worked, then we could continue to use them on the weekends and even when they left the residential care. I really wanted to know what they were doing, if it was working; I wanted to learn to use it. And they had four or five steps: crawling, and then you could walk, and then run, and then you could fly high. And those stood for how his behavior was doing. So, if he was "crawling," that means he was having a bad day, not following directions. And if he was "flying high" he had a really good day. It took me a while to figure it out because my explanation came from him. It was difficult for me because they continued to say, "We've never had a parent ask this before and want to be this involved." Why put him in a residential home. . . Stephen was there for a year-and-a-half, . . . and have staff do all these wonderful things with him, teach him different behaviors, how to cope, and then just send him home? Not teaching me what they discovered would be defeating the purpose of placement. He would likely end up right back there in a few weeks. Reluctantly, they began to work with me so that I could begin to incorporate some of these things at home. He was there for a year-and-a-half, and when it was getting close to the time for him to return home, we started to make the transition one step at a time. But I found out that this didn't happen in a lot of cases. When they felt like the child was ready to go home, they then set up a release date. And when the date was set, they would come to your home and talk to you about it a couple of times. But I wanted them to have a more extensive transition process for us. For one thing, Stephen moved into the group home before he entered public school. We had to realize this was a kid who had never been in a public school classroom, and he was coming home to a single mom with two other kids. This was going to be different for him. Most of the kids had been in public schools before placement in the residential home, and then were going back to a familiar setting. How could Stephen go into a classroom where there would be 25 or 30 children with one teacher, when all he's had is a special classroom in the residential home with five kids and three classroom teachers. He was used to the one-on-one tutoring. I knew that it would be a huge adjustment for him and for the teacher. Finally we had a meeting with the staff from the group home and some teachers at the school he was transitioning into, and we developed a plan for him to begin visiting the school. One of the staff from the residential center went with him. We started one week with him going to school just in the morning from eight to twelve, but it was over-whelming. There were 25 kids in the classroom, and he had to raise his hand before he spoke. None of this had to happen before because he had one-on-one teaching at the residential home. I thought that this was going to be a tough transition. Then for a week he went in the afternoons only. By the third week he went all day, but he still had a counselor from the residential home accompanying him all day.

It took three or four weeks to completely transition him into public school, but I think that was critical. At the same time he was spending more and more time at home. He would come on the weekend, but then he wouldn't go back until Tuesday, and so forth. There was a lot for him to get used to: going to school for the first time, and being home all the time . . . And I think that the transition period made it successful. But here again, this wasn't something that was initiated by the residential home. It is hard to duplicate the things they did at the center when he was at home. For example, Stephen has nightmares. One of the things they did in the group home was to set a desk and a chair right outside of Stephen's door, and they put a lamp on it so that a worker could do paperwork at night. If Stephen got afraid or had a nightmare, he knew that there was a worker sitting right at his door. I knew that this was happening because on the weekends Stephen ex-pected me to sleep or stand outside his door every night. And so I asked the group home to please wean him off of this because he really expected someone to be outside his door at home in case he became afraid. But they didn't want to do that. They didn't want him waking up with these nightmares and waking the other kids up. So they never did it. And it took forever at home for Stephen to sleep in his room by himself. If he woke up at home and I wasn't sitting outside his door, he would have little panic attacks. So one of the things that I continue to advocate for is to make sure that they are not putting the kids in situations that are impossible for families to keep up with at home. We didn't have shift workers at my house that could come in and sit up with him all night.

Because it is so structured at the residential home, they never gave the children independent time where they had to be on their own. They never sent them to their room to play by themselves or to be by themselves and create things to do to occupy their time. You know that in a home situation, kids need to know how to entertain themselves. They need to know how to go in their room to read a book or go put together a puzzle. And I found out that Stephen, because they structured every minute of his day, he didn't know how to entertain himself. When he came home, every thing he did, he needed to do it with Mom. "Ok, Mom, it's time for us to read a book." And even if I needed to fix dinner or do some housework, or help the girls with homework, . . . Stephen still expected to have me 24 hours a day, because when he was in the group home he had a worker 24 hours a day. I think that we can better prepare kids to return home and function in their family environment.

Interviewer: How would you evaluate the first placement in the near-by center?

Ms. Spencer: I'd probably put it right about a "B," because I think it was helpful to Stephen. It taught him better peer relationships–how to get along with other kids. It taught him a lot of self-control–controlling his anger and his temperament. They did teach me some things to use at home to help with his behavior. We had a few sessions with his sisters to teach them more about understanding what was going on with him. So I really thought that it helped. However, Stephen, in his own mind still sees it as "Mom gave me away. She abandoned me." So it's been hard for me to have him understand why he was there.

Interviewer: What was Stephen's diagnosis at the regional center?

Ms. Spencer: At the time, he had both an ADHD diagnosis and an

Oppositional Defiant Disorder Diagnosis, and he was on medications to treat those. But right before it was time for him to exit the group home, we really realized that he was bipolar. He was then about six years old and the medication was changed.

Interviewer: Did that help to stabilize things at home?

Ms. Spencer: It helped me to understand him better, but the medication didn't change his behaviors a whole lot. Even though the diagnosis was different, the medication wasn't changed much until recently.

Interviewer: Later there was another placement at a university hospital's in-patient psychiatric unit. How old was Stephen then?

Ms. Spencer: He was eight. There was a two-year span between the two.

Interviewer: What led up to this placement?

Ms. Spencer: The first one was when he was around four-and-a-half and we were really worried about getting him ready for school or being able to manage behaviors. He was diagnosed with a bipolar illness by the time he was eight because we were really starting to see severe mood swings from the depression and the manic behavior. And about October he started getting into a manic stage where he was extremely hyper, thoughts were racing, he was just having a horrible time focusing. He wasn't functioning in the classroom, and so we started to make some medication changes, just to bring him down from the mania. But it didn't work. He was having a horrible time at school and his psychiatrist was beginning to think that maybe the whole medication regimen wasn't right. There were just so many answers we didn't know. Then Stephen started to express some suicidal thoughts, and he started to do things that were questionable. We couldn't tell whether he was really making suicide attempts or not. We finally thought that he needed to be the hospitalized. It was a residential-type hospital treatment placement because they had the school and everything right there. It was a different experience because they talked, right from the beginning, about how they wanted the family to be involved. They didn't have rigid rules for visitations; they encouraged families to come. They had a library, and they encouraged us to look at videos and check out certain books about children's psychiatric disorders and disabilities.

The hospital is two-and-a-half hours away. It bothered me that Stephen would be so far away, but I felt a little better because he was older. It wasn't like leaving a four year old. The hospital connected me with the Ronald McDonald house so that I was able to visit and spend the night. I had to play "Super mom." I'd go visit him one day, then stay home two days and then go back. I did go up there about every three days. And they had it so that you could call anytime. They took him off all his medications because we had not taken a look at "Stephen" in quite a while, to see how he was without any medications. They confirmed the bipolar diagnosis and then they added on Obsessive-Compulsive Disorder.

That experience was somewhat better for me because I felt like I was a part of everything they did . . . they kept me informed. They called me, and there was a special time every day, when the doctors made their rounds, that the families could call and literally speak to the doctors and ask questions. They gave us a block of time to do that, and that made me feel a lot better. Every day I could find out what was going on. And whenever they changed a medication or added one . . . Whatever they did, they always called. When they got ready to discharge him from the hospital, I was pushing for a transition plan, but I think the distance made it more difficult. Before we knew it he was being discharged, and we had not put the transition plan in place. Altogether he was there about four weeks.

Interviewer: Would it have helped if he had been there longer?

Ms. Spencer: Oh, I'm sure, but this was one of those cases where insurance ran out and they said, "He's well. Take him home. It's been 30 days." That has been an issue for a lot of places. However, if the time limitation had not been a reality, would it have made more sense to have had a longer transition period? Yes, because they detoxed him, took him off all of his medications, and then they started to try different medicines. You know, it takes a long time to try a medication, get the dosage right to see it it's going to work. Well, they discharged him before they finished that process. So he came home and we were still playing around with dosages. And you could tell he wasn't completely well when he came home.

I tried to put him back in school. But he was so out of sorts the school said, "No. He can't come back." He was still really emotionally distraught. He'd cry at the drop of a hat. He'd gone over into a depression. He just wouldn't eat. It was just weird. So we came up with a plan so that he went to school a few hours a day and then came home. We ended up having to transition him here because the hospital was just too far away to take that on. It was really hard to try to get the different providers to communicate, and it was hard to get the psychiatrist here to talk regularly with the psychiatrist at the hospital. We lost some time and some consistency in his treatment because of the distance. But I think if we had worked out that transition piece with the hospital, it would've made it a better experience. The experience was pretty good, it was the transition that didn't go well.

How would I rate the university hospital placement? Well, probably an "A-minus." I guess one of the things that I was impressed with them about was that they looked at more of Stephen than just behaviors. Stephen was having problems with bed wetting, and they decided that was something they wanted to work on with him. They got this bell-pad, and they worked with him. They thought that was an important part of his life, too. It was a psychiatric unit, but they wanted to attend to other things.

They also wanted to help improve his relationships with his sisters because he has been having some problems with them. They encouraged me to bring his sisters on the visitation. The workers monitored how he played with them. They gave him some suggestions, and they were more family-centered with me. They wanted to pull in everybody and say, "Let's just see how this works." When I visited Stephen, I sensed that they really respected our relationship and our culture and the way we did things. They *asked* how we did things. They asked about our religious preferences. They asked permission for Stephen to participate in some religious services there since they knew we did that at home. And I had not had any cultural issues mentioned in the previous residential treatment placement, but the hospital staff was sensitive to that. It made me feel better. They even found a person from a local church that came and did activities with Stephen. That was important because one of the things Stephen missed when he was in the hospital was going to church and doing the things we did at home.

Interviewer: The readers of this journal are likely to be primarily psychiatrists, psychologists, social workers like myself, and other professionals who work at residential treatment centers. What recommendations would you make to them? Please consider the question from a broad viewpoint because you are the director of a family advocacy agency and know the experiences of other families.

Ms. Spencer: I tell parents, "When our kids were born with a serious mental or emotional challenge, they didn't come with a 'How-

To' manual." I mean, nobody gave me something that said, "This is how you raise a bipolar child." The people who work in these residential treatments have had years and years of advanced training on how to manage these kids. Sharing that kind of training and knowledge with family members is critical. Children in residential treatment settings learn wonderful ways to control their behaviors, and the staff should also teach the family new ways to respond when their child comes home. If the kid comes home and the family structure and interactions haven't changed, the kid will start to go back to old behaviors. That has happened to us at times . . . I get in a panic thinking, "Oh, he had stopped doing that. Why is he doing it again?!" And you start to blame yourself as a parent because you just don't know what to do. I watched some of the things they did when I would go visit Stephen. I would really watch the interaction because . . . one of the neat things about the university hospital was they had a room where the parents could watch the kids and the kids didn't know we were there. Well, I watched the way some of the workers interacted with him and how they got him to comply to certain rules. And I would think, "Wow. I hadn't tried that." I ended up with a whole list of things I try at home.

At the same time, they watched how I interacted with Stephen. This was really validating because there were some things that I was doing with Stephen that they thought were helpful. So we taught each other. There was a mutual respect. And that's something that we parents usually don't get. Usually we were told, "Everything you were doing was wrong and you shouldn't be doing that with your kid." But they really liked some of the ways that we interacted as a family and how Stephen had found his place in our family. That was one of the things I was able to share with them . . . One of the male workers in the hospital would say to Stephen, "Stephen, you're the man of the family. You're the only boy and you've got to be a man. You've got to take responsibility." Well, I said, "Stephen's problem is that he doesn't know how to take his place as a kid in my family. And although he doesn't have a dad living in the home, I'm the mom and that makes me the head of the family." I think Stephen really thought that because he was the only boy, that meant that he had to take on a lot of responsibility in our family, and I didn't want adults saying that to him. I would rather them say, "You are eight years old. You are a kid." Stephen would worry about where food was going to come from, or, "does mom have enough gas to take me to school?" And as he would worry, he would really get upset. Instead, I needed to reinforce, "You are the kid, and mom is going to figure out what's for supper tonight. Mom is going to take care of you." So that was one thing the hospital staff was able to learn from me; I had seen Stephen get so stressed and obsessive about wanting to make sure my family was taken care of, but he was only eight years old! The hospital staff listened to me and learned from my experience.

Mutual respect and believing that learning and discovery is two-ways, was helpful. Families need to be given a voice–what are their hopes, dreams, and aspirations? Then you try to help them get there. Even though their kids have special needs, you best believe that mom and dad have positive dreams for their child. It was helpful for me to see one of the workers tell Stephen, "Your mom says you are real smart in school, and that you love science. You can be a scientist. You can do something in science and you need to work hard." Well, that was something I had articulated about Stephen and it was good to see that they had picked up on the fact that we still have hopes and dreams for Stephen, even though Stephen was having a whole lot of challenges. Service providers need to listen to parents, follow their approach, and share their hopes and dreams; and then give them the training and support that they need to fulfill them.

One last thing to think about, and I don't know how confidentiality plays in this, but we've found that support groups have been really helpful for families. When they get together, they talk amongst themselves. It happened naturally for me when Stephen was in the university hospital. When I was there visiting my son I would meet other family members who were visiting. Somehow we would congregate and start talking, and it was so supportive. I wish that would happen as a planned activity in all residential placements . . . because it is a critical time for families–when their child is away from home. Why not plan a time when all the families could talk and support one another?

There was another lady who traveled quite a distance, as I did; but we didn't even realize we were both staying at the Ronald McDonald house! It was funny because we had both been there the whole week, and then right as we were leaving we realized that she was right down the hall from me. We could've really supported each other, both of us having our kids in the child psychiatric unit at the same time.

Are we still in the old days when it was believed that mental illness should be hidden instead of just saying, "This is just a fact of life that can occur to almost anyone, and there is no blame!" Perhaps we need to get families together to share experiences and gain support from one another, but it's just something I haven't seen residential centers do. The residential treatment staff could serve as facilitators and resource people. Also, some families might like to be assigned a mentor or a special family support person who has been through the experience. Whenever you go through this, you just don't even realize that hundreds of people have gone through it, because it is so personal to you and it hurts so much. If someone was there to say, "My kid was in this hospital ten years ago and he's fine now, and our family is okay now, and we will help you get through it, too." Something like that would have been really helpful.

BIOGRAPHICAL NOTE

Ms. Sandra Spencer is a graduate of East Carolina University with a degree in English and Communications. To be certain that her son's mental health needs were adequately met, she developed advocacy skills. She soon discovered that there were many other children with serious emotional disturbances whose mental health needs were not being addressed, and she, therefore, organized an advocacy, support group for families called WE-CARE (With Every Child and Adult Reaching Excellence). She has become nationally recognized for her leadership, and travels extensively speaking on behalf of children with serious emotional disturbances and their families. Recently she testified before the US Congress, and urged its members to address the urgent need for comprehensive and quality community-based and family-centered children's mental health services.

"A Matter of Economics"

The nomadic ten-year old
Who had traveled many streets,
Listening to a different beat
Or maybe searching for his own

Could not, or would not, adapt
To the current token economy
Whereby he had to do good,
A priori, to receive attention.

Good acts had to be observed
Directly, by the paymasters.
At his negative manifestations
The paymasters turned away.

He tried reporting good things,
Good thoughts to them every day:
But seeing is believing,
Second-hand is not negotiable.

They turned away so much, until
He thought they'd break their necks,
Or half-way wished they would.
And then wished all the way.

But I keep on wishing that someone
Could like me once, just for me.
When you have to pay ahead of time
It takes all the fun away.

Douglas Powers, MD

[Haworth co-indexing entry note]: "A Matter of Economics." Powers, Douglas. Co-published simultaneously in *Residential Treatment for Children & Youth* (The Haworth Press, Inc.) Vol. 17, No. 3, 2000, p. 45; and: *Family-Centered Services in Residential Treatment: New Approaches for Group Care* (ed: John Y. Powell) The Haworth Press, Inc., 2000, p. 45. Single or multiple copies of this article are available for a fee from The Haworth Document Delivery Service [1-800-342-9678, 9:00 a.m. - 5:00 p.m. (EST). E-mail address: getinfo@haworthpressinc.com].

45

The Carolinas Project:
A Comprehensive Intervention
to Support Family-Centered
Group Care Practice

Floyd J. Alwon, EdD
Laurie A. Cunningham, BA
James Phills, PhD
Andrew L. Reitz, PhD
Richard W. Small, PhD
Virginia M. Waldron, MEd

SUMMARY. The child welfare system continues its challenge to find better ways for achieving safe permanent connections between children, youths and their families. The importance of maintaining these relationships, especially when children have been removed from their families for periods of time, has been consistently substantiated in the literature (Braziel, 1996; Pecora, Whittaker & Maluccio, 1992; Wells, Wyatt, & Hobfoll, 1991). However, many residential providers, particularly those with long histories as orphanages and children's homes, have been reluctant to embrace family-centered practices as these are often perceived to conflict with their historical, child-rescue missions (see Table 1).

The authors wish to acknowledge The Duke Endowment and the departments of social services in North and South Carolina for their support for this project. Mr. Robert A. Mayer, II is especially acknowledged for his vision, leadership and steadfast commitment to keeping children and families connected.

The authors may be written at Walker Trieschman Center, 300 Congress Street, Suite 305, Quincey, MA 02169.

[Haworth co-indexing entry note]: "The Carolinas Project: A Comprehensive Intervention to Support Family-Centered Group Care Practice." Alwon, Floyd J. et al. Co-published simultaneously in *Residential Treatment for Children & Youth* (The Haworth Press, Inc.) Vol. 17, No. 3, 2000, pp. 47-62; and: *Family-Centered Services in Residential Treatment: New Approaches for Group Care* (ed: John Y. Powell) The Haworth Press, Inc., 2000, pp. 47-62. Single or multiple copies of this article are available for a fee from The Haworth Document Delivery Service [1-800-342-9678, 9:00 a.m. - 5:00 p.m. (EST). E-mail address: getinfo@haworthpressinc.com].

Some providers who have attempted to move toward more family-centered residential care have found it necessary to confront a lack of support from the service systems in which they operate. Other organizations, however, have been able to make extraordinary progress in reinventing their treatment philosophy and services (Gruenwald, 1996). Not surprisingly, the leadership in these settings strongly supported the changes and helped to secure the extra resources needed to facilitate strategic change (Kanter, Stein, & Jick, 1992; Kotter, 1990; Nadler & Tushman, 1989). This article describes a unique strategic change intervention designed to help a large number of residential providers in North and South Carolina become more family-centered. The article also reports on the project's outcomes and outlines lessons learned from this experience.

The Duke Endowment of Charlotte, North Carolina has provided direct and indirect support to residential child caring agencies in North and South Carolina since 1924. The Group Child Care Consultant Services of the University of North Carolina at Chapel Hill and the state trade associations, longtime beneficiaries of this endowment, helped many of these programs in their initial transition from orphanage/children's home to a more treatment-oriented approach.

The Child Care Division of The Duke Endowment under the leadership of Robert Mayer, was committed to strengthening family-centered practice. The Endowment had previously funded an initiative whose efforts focused on enhancing family-centered competence among clinically-oriented staff. In 1993, in response to a request for a proposal, the Albert E. Trieschman Center submitted a plan to provide training and technical assistance to help residential providers in North and South Carolina become more family-centered. This multi-year project, The Carolinas Project, initially featured a comprehensive staff development program with an accompanying technical assistance component. The project later focused on facilitating closer collaboration between private providers and public agencies. The Trieschman Center, a Massachusetts based, national resource center, helps practitioners find better ways of working with high risk children, youth, and families.[1] *[Article copies available for a fee from The Haworth Document Delivery Service: 1-800-342-9678. E-mail address: getinfo@ haworthpressinc.com <Website: http://www.haworthpressinc.com>]*

KEYWORDS. Family-centered group care, intervention, training

CAROLINAS PROJECT DESCRIPTION

The primary goals of The Carolinas Project (TCP) were to help staff in residential child care facilities become more receptive to working with family members; to increase staff competence in working with families; to support facilities modifications to assure a more family-friendly milieu; and to facilitate dialogue between providers and public agency staff. The proposed workplan was reviewed with input from a national advisory board and regional steering committees.

Phase I

A modified plan for what later became known as Phase I began in early 1994. Early goals for project staff included establishing relationships and credibility with influential leaders; developing curricula for training and technical assistance; and devising a program evaluation model. Hiring a Carolinas-based coordinator with a strong commitment to family-centered work clearly became a critical component in the overall success of this project.

In an effort to clarify the philosophical rationale supporting family-centered practice, a "working paper" was widely distributed. This paper, modified later for publication (Ainsworth & Small, 1995), offered the following definition of family-centered group care practice:

TABLE 1. From Child-Centered to Family-Centered Group Care Practice

	Child-Centered Group Care	Family-Centered Group Care
Focus	Child welfare.	Family and child welfare.
Reason for out-of-home care	Poor parenting. Parental neglect. Parental abuse.	Family stress, environmental and psychological, limited adaptation and coping skills.
Intervention	Protect child by separation from parents. Treat parents and/or remove parental rights.	Protect child as necessary but recognize parents' continuing place in the child's life and accept them as equal partners in the child rearing process.
How parents are viewed	Blame them for their inadequacy.	Support parents' efforts to make positive contributions to their child's life.
Child & youth care tasks	Look after children until they grow up, if necessary.	Teach parents wherever possible how to look after their own children. If not possible, maintain active connections between parent and child throughout period of child's out-of-home care.

Table 1 adapted from Hansen & Ainsworth (1983). Family and parenting analogies in Australian residential child care. *Australian Child and Family Welfare, 8,3/4,3-5.*

Family-centered practice in group care settings is characterized by a set of institutional structures and a range of services, supports and professional practices designed to preserve and, whenever possible, to strengthen connections between each child in placement and his or her family. Whether the function of the group care setting is to provide short-term shelter, longer term care, or residential treatment, a primary goal of placement is always to work toward each child's optimum involvement in family life, even in situations where full-time reunification is not possible.

The paper also included a listing of practice principles (see Table 2). This allowed potential project participants to begin to reflect on their organization's level of family-centered practice.

Project staff also gave presentations on this subject at statewide conferences. Residential agencies historically assisted by The Duke Endowment were invited to participate in this project. Thirty-seven agencies agreed to contribute a nominal fee as a sign of their commitment (three additional agencies joined the project at a later date). Project staff then grouped agencies into geographical clusters, assigned a consultant to each agency, and scheduled the training/consultation cycles.

The project coordinator made a site visit to each agency to introduce the project in further detail, to address concerns and to describe the Trieschman Family Centered Group Care Instrument (TFCGCI). This self-assessment instrument was designed to measure an organization's level of family-centered practice in four areas: family participation in program; family involvement in decision making;

TABLE 2. Basic Principles of Family-Centered Group Care Practice

- Placement can be both child-centered and family-affirming.
- Group care is not necessarily the choice of last resort.
- Children and families are irrevocably linked.
- All families have potential.
- Family-centered practice promotes family empowerment and builds on strengths.
- Family-centered practice respects family diversity.
- Family-centered practice requires flexible teamwork.
- Family-centered practice requires maximum feasible contact.

Table 2 adapted from Maluccio, Warsh, & Ing, 1993 and from Ainsworth & Small 1995 availability of services to families; and staff attitudes to families (Ainsworth, 1997). The instrument was completed by all staff at each agency. A research team entered the data and generated a report for each organization. The TFCGCI served to introduce the values and beliefs underlying the project in a non-threatening manner. A consultant visited each agency prior to the training cycle to review the results of the TFCGCI and to address questions or concerns. The training intervention began shortly thereafter.

Each organization enrolled staff members representing all positions, including direct care, supervisory, support, clinical, and executive for trainings offered in eight regional clusters throughout the two states. The curriculum began with a half-day orientation for all staff and continued for approximately two months. The orientation session highlighted the principles underlying this project and presented information about organizational change. Following the orientation, direct care staff (child care workers, houseparents, social workers, and their supervisors), participated in three full-days of training; supervisors received an additional full-day; and support staff, one half-day. CEOs participated in informal discussion groups for one half-day at the beginning and another at the end of the training cycle. The sessions for supervisors and administrators focused on helping them to support their staff during the change process.

The curriculum was developed based on adult education principles and methodology. The learning objectives include a substantial emphasis on attitude. Participants were encouraged to explore their personal beliefs and prejudices and to examine how their organization's policies and practices affected family-centered practice. A participant action plan component was deployed to support transfer of learning to the work site.

During the one-year intervention, a consultant with expertise in family-centered programming worked with a steering committee from each organization to support their efforts to develop and complete an agencywide action plan. Each organization received approximately six days of individualized consultation and technical assistance. The consultant assigned to each organization typically delivered four days of consultation following completion of the training intervention. The consultant's charge was loosely prescribed given the differences among agencies in size, resources, states of readiness, etc. The consultant negotiated his/her involvement with the administrator and the agency's steering committee. Common activities for consultants included making presentations to boards of directors; reviewing program literature such as policy and procedure manuals; assisting with the development of family orientation handbooks; and providing consultation on proposed architectural plans.

A closing session served as the graduation ritual for each regional cluster. Representatives from each participating organization along with key project staff attended this special meeting. At this meeting, program staff shared their accomplishments and, to some degree, their ongoing challenges.

Additional activities associated with Phase I included the creation of a newsletter designed to highlight promising practices taking place throughout the Carolinas. Project staff also helped to plan a special conference jointly sponsored by the child care associations from both states. The conference, the first such joint venture undertaken by these associations, attracted more than 400 participants with a conference theme–"All in the Family."

Phase II

Based on progress noted during Phase I, The Duke Endowment decided to support recommendations from the project's steering committee to expand the scope of the project through a second phase to begin January, 1997. Activities from both phases ran concurrently for approximately one year because several of the regionally based trainings had not yet completed their twelve-month cycle. All but one agency from Phase I opted to participate in Phase II.

A primary goal for the two-year period of Phase II was to increase collaboration in family-centered service provision between participating care providers and the public sector (most specifically, county and regional offices of the departments of social services). Additional goals included: offering ongoing basic training for new staff;. providing more advanced training in family-centered practice; implementing a training-for-trainers process; supporting continued collaboration among private providers; and producing an enhanced newsletter.

Phase II activities, more numerous and generally broader in scope than those associated with Phase I, included five components: The Public/Private Partnership Program; Family Focused Forums; Core Curriculum Training; Training for Trainers; and The Carolinas Project Newsletter.

Public/Private Partnership

This component brought together representatives from providers who participated in Phase I and public sector organizations responsible for child placement. Counties whose departments of social services included the largest number of children in out-of home placement were targeted as primary participants, although participation by smaller counties and other public sector agencies such as the Guardian Ad Litem program and the juvenile court system was also welcomed.

Caseworkers and their supervisors were the primary participants from the public sector, while private sector agencies were represented by a cross-section of staff. A regional clustering, similar to that used in Phase I, was implemented. In total, twelve geographic clusters of public and private organizations participated over the two-year period. Participants attended a day-long session in a format best described as facilitated interactions between public and private sector representatives. The discussion focused on family-centered practice and explored collaborative service provision specific to the communities represented. Participants identified needs and developed action plans.

Voluntary task groups were formed to continue addressing identified issues. A project consultant was assigned to each task group to provide ongoing support and technical assistance. Leadership for these groups was drawn from the group itself, with co-chairs representing public and private sectors. Task force groups were formed on a county-specific basis or regionally, based on the needs and wishes of each group. A total of ten task force groups were formed with half continuing to meet at the close of the project. Projects undertaken by task force groups include initiating quarterly networking and training sessions; revising referral and intake processes to facilitate more timely and complete sharing of case information; and creating a more effective collaborative case planning process.

Family-Focused Forums

Family-focused forums were designed to enhance skills developed during the initial phase of TCP, to give and receive consultative feedback on challenging cases, and to provide participating organizations with continued support for their family-centered initiatives. These one-day forums took place quarterly in geographically accessible regions. Examples of topics addressed include: joining with families; assessing families; goal setting; networking with the public sector; and working with hard-to-reach families. Project staff co-facilitated these sessions with presenters who had topic expertise.

Core Curriculum Training

A three-day condensed version of the project's core curriculum was offered regionally in both states several times per year. Consumers included several provider organizations that did not participate in Phase I as well as new employees from agencies that had participated in Phase I.

Training for Trainers

A training for trainers program was devised to develop local capacity to continue offering the core curriculum upon completion of the project. Prospective trainers attended the core curriculum training and then remained on site for two additional days of instruction in the principles of adult education, with special reference to its application in teaching the project's curriculum. They then co-trained a future course and received coaching and feedback from project staff.

Newsletter

The newsletter significantly expanded in scope and quality during Phase II. What began as a simple project update designed for internal use developed into a vehicle that featured promising practices and resource information from the Carolinas but also from around the country. Project staff were positively impressed by the number of submissions for publication by project participants.

PROJECT OUTCOMES

Assessing outcomes for a complex, multi-year project involving hundreds of participants from diverse organizational settings is no simple matter. Nonetheless, evaluators identified numerous indicators of success, most especially in Phase I. These include: process outcomes such as the development of a comprehensive, well-tested curriculum, changes in staff knowledge and attitude and substantial modification of agency practice in relation to families.

Evaluation data were collected to assess each of the above outcomes. Participant evaluations of the project training curriculum were consistently high throughout the project. The revised 3-day training program used during Phase II received the highest ratings. Pre-post measures also indicated that the training resulted in significant improvements in staff knowledge regarding family-centered care and in their attitudes toward working collaboratively with family members. Finally, the data from the second administration of the TFCGCI and the agency action plans indicate that the project had a significant impact on actual agency practice. TFCGCI data showed that agencies made significant improvements in the levels of parent involvement and decision making in their programs, as well as in the overall availability of services directly targeting families and family members. In addition, agencies achieved a large number of specific goals targeted in the action planning process. Some of these outcomes, corroborated by the project consultants, include:

- 70% created or revised a family-friendly admissions handbook.
- 25% established a parent advisory committee, or added parent(s) to the governing board.
- 30% made significant policy changes to create a more family-friendly environment.
- 30% produced newsletters for families.
- 15% built new structures or remodeled existing buildings to provide services for families.

The process of securing endorsement for a set of Indicators of Family-Centered Group Care Practice served as a unifying activity, one that helped to pull together the thinking among the leadership of the Regional Steering Committee. Project staff culled a limited number of proposed indicators from the project's Principles and the self assessment instrument. Project participants provided feedback with the Steering Committee having the most significant influence on the selection of the final set of indicators (see Table 3).

Evaluating Phase II is more difficult because some of the activities were not yet completed at the time of this writing. Initial results from participant assessment of knowledge and attitude gains in the family-centered forums (the more advanced skill-building sessions) and the public/private training sessions closely match those of Phase I. Feedback on enhancements to the project's newsletter has also been quite positive and distribution has been substantially increased to include the public sector.

Enrollment for the training sessions in Phase II, however, has been uneven across geographical regions. Project staff have struggled to increase attendance with varying degrees of success. The buy-in of a key leader in the local office of the department of social services clearly had positive impact on attendance. Yet, despite serious advanced marketing efforts, including face-to-face meetings between the project coordinator and the local office leadership, this commitment did not come easily and, even in those jurisdictions where the leadership supported the goals of the project, case crises often seriously restricted attendance. The outcomes from this component of Phase II will undoubtedly fall short of those achieved in the earlier phase. However, this could also be due to the fact that the intensity of the public sector intervention (e.g., hours of training) did not match the multiple exposures to the project's principles that was available to private sector participants in Phase I.

There was a noted shift in public policy on a national and local level away from the prior emphasis on preservation of families. State and county child welfare agencies began to expect that children would be removed from their families and placed in "more permanent homes" within a one-year period of being removed from their family of origin. These changes were also supported by print and electronic media that highlighted reports of abuse received by children who were returned

TABLE 3. Indicators of Family-Centered Practice

- Parents are provided with a handbook or materials, written specifically for them, that outlines relevant agency policies.
- An established, documented grievance procedure is in place for parents who have concerns about their child's care.
- Parents are recognized as full partners in the care of their child with equal input into planning and day-to-day decision making; and diligent efforts are made to insure parents' attendance at and/or participation in all meetings where decisions are made.
- There is a plan for regular and frequent communication between the agency and parents.
- Visiting and communication between children and their families is open, flexible and restricted as necessary only on a case-by-case basis.
- The agency extends assistance to families for whom a lack of resources prevents communication or contact.
- The agency provides for family visiting in privacy, in a space conducive to positive family interaction.
- Parents are represented on the Board and/or participate in a formal advisory process in order to provide input into agency policies, practices and program evaluation.
- The agency regularly solicits feedback from its consumers, including clients, families and referral sources.
- The agency works collaboratively with other service providers to families.

to their families. While difficult to measure, there is little doubt that these changes made it more difficult to maintain the progress achieved earlier in this project.

Leaders among private providers and public agencies in several regions report satisfactory experiences with the structured facilitation provided by project consultants. These consultants provide support services in arranging periodic meetings that address issues identified as obstacles to enhanced family-centered practices.

LESSONS LEARNED

Throughout the course of this undertaking, project staff met regularly to review progress and, where possible, made adjustments to the interventions to assure that the project met its stated goal of helping to strengthen connections between children in group care and families. The unique and complex nature of this project did not allow for any "cookbook" formula. Each provider organization and each CEO began at different levels of readiness and there were substantial differences in receptivity among the regional offices of the public agencies. Finally, one state has a county-driven system while the other is more centralized. Although the project is ongoing at the time of this writing, several lessons have been learned regarding the design of such large-scale change interventions.

Orientation to Core Values and Principles

During the first training cycle of Phase I, it became clear that project staff had overestimated the level of awareness and level of commitment to the project by many participants. In response, staff developed and distributed an orientation packet prior to the initial site-visit by the project coordinator. The packet included a cover letter, a curriculum summary, and a list of activities and handouts the administration could use to prepare staff for the work ahead. Project staff noted substantial improvement in participant readiness although a significant number of staff continued to arrive unprepared for the training experience.

Sharing core values and principles is an important first step in generating buy-in when developing collaborative initiatives (Shauffer & Soler,

1990; Simpson, 1998). As mentioned earlier, this was accomplished through distributing the working paper and the organizational self-assessment instrument (TFCGCI). These vehicles served to disseminate the core values for this project and helped to concretize the proposed intervention, providing specific areas in which to address one's concerns.

Resistance

In general, participants demonstrated more resistance to family-centered practice principles than anticipated. Project staff modified the curriculum before the end of the first training cycle in an attempt to address this issue. These revisions included the addition of more empathy building activities in an attempt to facilitate attitudinal changes among participants. An activity was also added that acknowledged that a substantial number of trainees resented the fact that the training was mandated by their organization. These changes appeared to enhance positive participation.

Need for Direction

Early in the consultation process a few CEOs expressed the need for more direction from their consultant. They felt that staff and consultants were overly deferential to the feelings of agency administrators and not prescriptive enough about what was or was not family-centered practice. This initial approach undoubtedly reflected consultants' attempts to appear sensitive to regional and organizational values. Consultants modified future interventions to be more prescriptive as needed.

Role of Motivation

Motivation plays an obvious critical role in determining the success of change interventions (Beer, Eisenstat & Spector, 1990; Kanter, 1985). A graduate class from a prestigious business school studied The Carolinas Project proposal and determined that there was little chance of success for this intervention. They based their findings on several factors. Making strategic change in one organization is difficult enough; making change in multiple settings seemed too ambitious especially given the limited resources available for this undertaking.

Most importantly, they noted the absence of perceived urgency. The residential providers overall were doing well with their occupancy rates and had experienced little internal or external pressure to become more family-centered in their practice. Organizations typically only make significant change under duress, when it is clear that "the wolf is at the door." The powerful force of inertia must be overcome before change can occur (Hanna & Freeman, 1984; Lawler & Galbraith, 1994).

With the benefit of hindsight, this assessment by the business students neglected to understand the powerful influence of The Duke Endowment. Invitations to participate in the project came from the Endowment, an organization that has provided generous support to these residential providers for many years. The director of the foundation's child care division had close relationships with the CEOs from these organizations and his presence at the project's meetings and trainings clearly helped to "bring folks to the table." Several CEOs acknowledged making the transition from initial skepticism to commitment.

CEO Involvement

The support of the chief executive officer is generally considered a "critical success factor" in strategic change (Kotter, 1995; Nutt & Backoff, 1993). The absence of active CEO participation undermined the impact of the training in some organizations. Participants frequently mentioned that they felt their directors should be present at more of the training sessions. Not surprisingly, organizations were generally more successful in meeting goals when the administration embraced the project and demonstrated visibility at the training sessions. Similarly, agencies that had multiple "champions" for family-centered practice also made more immediate and noteworthy gains.

Peer Influence

Peer influence played a significant role in supporting the project's goals, even more so than originally anticipated. The project provided a number of networking opportunities for residential providers during Phase I and later in Phase II with their public agency colleagues. At these meetings, it was not uncommon to observe positive peer influence, particularly among CEOs, many of whom had previously developed relationships from other arenas. The strengthening of collaborative relationships, a positive by-product of this project, has the potential to continue to enhance outcomes for children and families in the Carolinas. These organizations are well-positioned to pool their resources for staff development activities and to begin to develop community based services and service networks, activities typically associated with managed care.

Multiple Exposures/Facets

This project clearly underlined the need for a comprehensive and well-coordinated series of interventions to produce significant change. These interventions included an orientation program, a core training curricula, specialized training, and a technical assistance component. Perhaps the most important lesson learned from this undertaking is the need to provide multiple exposures to a core set of critical themes that support the project's primary goals–helping to keep children and families connected.

NOTE

1. The Albert E. Trieschman Center was a division of The Walker Home and School until July 1, 1998 at which point the Trieschman Center continued its management of The Carolinas Project as the Walker Trieschman Center, a division of the Child Welfare League of America.

REFERENCES

Ainsworth, F. (1997). *Family Centered Group Care: Model Building.* Aldershot: Ashgate.
Ainsworth, F., Malucio, A.N., & Small, R.W. (1996). A framework for family-centered group care practice: Guiding principles and practice implications. In D.J. Braziel (Ed.), *Family-Focused Practice in Out-of-Home Care.* Washington, DC: Child Welfare League of America.
Ainsworth, F., & Small, R.W. (1995). Family-centered group care practice: Concept and implementation. *Journal of Child and Youth Care Work,* 7-14.
Ainsworth, F., Small, R.W., & Hanson, P. (1994). *The Carolinas Project Instrument.* Needham, MA: Albert E. Trieschman Center.
Beer, M., Eisenstat, R., & Spector, B. (1990). Why change programs don't produce change. *Harvard Business Review,* 68(6), 158-166.
Braziel, D.J. (Ed.), (1996). *Family-Focused Practice in Out-of-Home Care.* Washington, DC: Child Welfare League of America.
Gruenewald, A. (1996). Integrating family-focused practice into out-of-home care

In D.J. Braziel (Ed.), *Family-Focused Practice in Out-of-Home Care*. Washington, DC: Child Welfare League of America.

Hannan, M.T., & Freeman, J. (1984). Structural inertia and organizational change. *American Sociological Review*, 49(2), 149-164.

Hansen, P. & Ainsworth, F. (1983). Family and parenting analogies in Australian residential child care. *Australian Child and Family Welfare*, 8, 3/4, 3-5.

Kanter, R.M. (1985). Managing the human side of change. *Management Review*, 74(4), 52-56.

Kanter, R.M., Stein, B.A., & Jick, T.D. (Eds.) (1992). *The Challenge of Organizational Change: How Companies Experience It and Leaders Guide It*. New York: Free Press.

Kotter, J.P. (1990). *A Force for Change: How Leadership Differs from Management*. New York: Free Press.

Kotter, J.P. (1995). Leading change: Why transformation efforts fail. *Harvard Business Review*, 73(2), 59-68.

Lawler, E.E., & Galbraith, J.R. (1994). Avoiding the corporate dinosaur syndrome. *Organizational Dynamics*, 23(2), 5-17.

Maluccio, A.N., Warsh, R., & Pine, B.A. (1993). Family reunification: An overview. In B.A. Pine, R. Warsh, & A.N. Maluccio (Eds.), *Together Again: Family Reunification in* Foster Care. Washington, DC: Child Welfare League of America.

Nadler, D.A., & Tuchman, M.L. (1989). Organizational frame bending: Principles for managing reorientation. *Academy of Management Executive*, 3(3), 194-204.

Nutt, P.C., & Backoff, R.W. (1993). Transforming public organizations with strategic management and strategic leadership. *Journal of Management*, 19(2), 299-347.

Pecora, P.J., Whittaker, J.K., & Maluccio, A.N. (1992). *The Child Welfare Challenge: Policy, Practice, and Research*. New York: Aldine De Gruyter.

Shauffer, C., & Soler, M. (1990) Fighting fragmentation: Coordination of services for children and families. *Nebraska Law Review*, 69, 278-285.

Simpson, Jr., C.E. (1998). Increasing capabilities through coalitions. *Closing the Gap*, Newsletter of Office of Minority Health Resource Center, US Department of Health and Human Services, April, p.3.

Wells, K., Wyatt, E., & Hobfoll, S. (1991). Factors associated with adaptation of youth discharged from residential treatment. *Children and Youth Services Review*, 13, 199-216.

BIOGRAPHICAL NOTES

Floyd J. Alwon, EdD, director of professional development and the Walker Trieschman Center, Child Welfare League of America, has thirty years experience in child welfare, special education, and behavioral health. Dr. Alwon began his career as a child care worker and has also served as a supervisor, administrator, trainer, and consultant. He served as project director for The Carolinas Project.

Andy Reitz, PhD, is a clinical psychologist with more than 25 years experience in programs serving children and families. He has worked as a welfare caseworker, high school teacher, child care worker, supervisor, therapist, university instructor, program director, and agency administrator. He is currently employed as a private consultant and as a senior associate at the Walker Trieschman Center of the Child Welfare League of America. Dr. Reitz served as a consultant to several participating organizations in The Carolinas Project.

Ginnie Waldron, MEd, has more than 25 years experience in the area of child welfare. She has served as a child care worker, supervisor, and director of residential services. Currently, the director of training for the Walker Trieschman Center of the Child Welfare League of America, She served as project manager, consultant and trainer for The Carolinas Project.

Laurie Cunningham has more than 20 years experience in child welfare primarily working with at-risk youth and their families. She worked as a social worker in both the public and private sectors and currently as an independent consultant and trainer. She was project coordinator and senior trainer for The Carolinas Project.

Richard Small, PhD, has served as the executive director of the Walker Home and School since 1985. He is an author, educator, and consultant to child welfare programs around the world. He also served as executive director of the Massachusetts Governor's Advisory Committee on Child and the Family. Dr. Small served as a consultant and primary writer of curricula for The Carolinas Project.

James Phills, PhD, is Associate Professor at the School of Management at Yale University. He has written and consulted widely on strategic change and organizational development. He has served on the board of directors of The Walker Home and School and on the advisory committee of the Trieschman Center.

"The Bishop Visits"

Christine, in her bubbly,
Friendly, directly affronting,
Completely uninhibited,
Frequently disorganized way,

Ran swiftly across the grounds
Toward the visiting Bishop,
To the great astonishment
Of his hierarchical entourage,

Yelling at the top of her voice,
I know what's wrong with him:
The Bishop has fleas,
The Bishop has fleas.

Now almost anyone knows
That there are no flies
On no Bishops at no time,
And certainly no fleas.

But the Bishop knew
Just what to do,
And on bended knee
In the green grass
He and Christine
Exchanged quiet information
About collars: clerical,
Canine, and otherwise.

[Haworth co-indexing entry note]: "The Bishop Visits." Powers, Douglas. Co-published simultaneously in *Residential Treatment for Children & Youth* (The Haworth Press, Inc.) Vol. 17, No. 3, 2000, pp. 63-64; and: *Family-Centered Services in Residential Treatment: New Approaches for Group Care* (ed: John Y. Powell) The Haworth Press, Inc., 2000, pp. 63-64. Single or multiple copies of this article are available for a fee from The Haworth Document Delivery Service [1-800-342-9678, 9:00 a.m. - 5:00 p.m. (EST). E-mail address: getinfo@haworthpressinc.com].

And now Christine knows
As everyone knows
That Bishops are not,
Repeat, not infested.

Christine also knows that dogs
Wearing white collars are not,
Necessarily, Canines of the Cloth
And she likes having a new friend.

Douglas Powers, MD

Joining Family-Centered Care
and the Team Approach:
A Conversation About the Process

Rebecca S. Barboff, MS
M. Theresa Palmer, MSW
Meribeth Robinson, MS
Larry B. Sharpe, MSW

SUMMARY. The following conversation took place on May 29, 1998. This dialogue provided an opportunity to reflect on the tremendous changes that have taken place at The Children's Home, Inc., a residential facility founded in 1909, as it has evolved from custodial care to a systemic, family-centered program offering a broad continuum of services. Topics range from the pain and trauma of change to the excitement and tremendous sense of accomplishment that intertwine themselves throughout this process.

The four staff members involved in the discussion have worked in a variety of positions in the residential field and, together, represent over 50 years of professional experience. (A brief profile of each person is located at the end of the discussion.) *[Article copies available for a fee from The Haworth Document Delivery Service: 1-800-342-9678. E-mail address: getinfo@haworthpressinc.com <Website: http://www.haworthpressinc.com>]*

Rebecca: When we first talked about writing an article for the journal *Residential Treatment for Children & Youth*, the thing that came to mind first was the major shift The

---

The authors may be written at The Children's Home, 1001 Reynolds Road, Winston-Salem, NC 27104-3200.

[Haworth co-indexing entry note]: "Joining Family-Centered Care and the Team Approach: A Conversation About the Process." Barboff, Rebecca S. et al. Co-published simultaneously in *Residential Treatment for Children & Youth* (The Haworth Press, Inc.) Vol. 17, No. 3, 2000, pp. 65-76; and: *Family-Centered Services in Residential Treatment: New Approaches for Group Care* (ed: John Y. Powell) The Haworth Press, Inc., 2000, pp. 65-76. Single or multiple copies of this article are available for a fee from The Haworth Document Delivery Service [1-800-342-9678, 9:00 a.m. - 5:00 p.m. (EST). E-mail address: getinfo@haworthpressinc.com].

Children's Home underwent as team and family-centered work began to emerge.

Larry: I agree. Some very good things came out of that shift but it also was a long, hard struggle. I believe we have some thing important to share with other people–with other agencies. There are things we might have done different ly, some lessons we learned painfully, that may help others get to the same outcome by a quicker route. It may be possible to contribute to that process by sharing our experiences.

Theresa: It also seems we're in the midst of a paradigm shift occurring within the residential field itself. Residential facilities are finding it harder and harder to operate independently from their surrounding communities. The shift to team- and family-centered work helped *us* integrate more with others–our work with their work. If we were going to practice systemically we had to reach out, interact, collaborate.

Meribeth: That's right. Forming partnerships with people in the community, even with families, had not been one of our biggest strengths. In fact, we used to be proud of our self-sufficiency–that everything was right here on campus! The Children's Home had been a custodial care facility for many years and we did that well. We knew how to take care of kids and provide a home for them that was a safe, caring, learning, nurturing environment. They grew up here–this was home for many many kids. Those kids were taught life skills like dairy farming, canning, growing foods, and so on.

Theresa: It might be helpful if we give a little background infomation on The Children's Home–sort of a short history. It'll be interesting to get Meribeth and Larry's perspective since they were here during the shift to family- and team-centered work.

Rebecca: And with two different perspectives–Larry in a clinical or administrative position and Meribeth as a direct care worker. So, where to begin.

Larry: Well, a lot of people think we used to be an orphanage but we never were. Although orphans and half-orphans lived here, there were kids from other family situations too. Like Meribeth mentioned earlier, the best term for what we did back then was "custodial care." In the early to mid-part of the century, we had 400 kids here at any one time. That changed and by the time I came here in 1982, the numbers gradually had come down to less than a hundred–operating somewhere around eighty children. Even this number was large, though, because events were planned for the entire campus at one time. We would load up all the kids to go on activities. We went in *large* groups and took trips on a big yellow school bus.

Rebecca: So was there a school here at that time?

Larry: Not then, but we had an old yellow school bus! And it would break down half way to wherever we were going.

Meribeth: We got rid of that bus shortly after I started working here. But we still did things with large groups of kids.

Larry: Yes, but the numbers continued to drop. At one point, we reached the low sixties–compared with four hundred a few decades before. With that shift in numbers came the recognition that "something's not happening–something is wrong." We began to realize that people and things had to change. The numbers continued to decrease as the types of problems children were experiencing be came more extreme. We were set up to do custodial care–not as a treatment facility. So, when children were placed here and didn't behave, we discharged them. It became a re-volving door. These unplanned discharges created a lot of discomfort because we weren't used to seeing kids leave prematurely and it wasn't a comfortable feeling.

Theresa: It must have been a painful experience to realize that what you'd done well for so long wasn't working any more and, as an organization, go about finding what to put in its place.

Rebecca: When do you think this realization began to occur–when did the types of problems children brought with them begin to change?

Larry: I'd say the 1960's and 70's–when the culture began to change rapidly. But it wasn't until the 1980's that we began to realize custodial care wasn't meeting these kids needs–that we had to begin working with their *families*.

Meribeth: That's right. When I came here in the mid-1980's as a direct care worker, staffing patterns were just beginning to change. This was really a good thing though! For example, it used to be hard on Christmas or Thanksgiving, when the entire campus would close. If kids didn't have a place to go, they would all be taken to the infirmary and spend their holiday there! The kids that were sent home were just dropped off or sent on a Greyhound bus. We had very little contact with families–next to none.

Larry: But again, the kinds of problems began to change–drugs, sexual abuse, violence–and we realized we couldn't address them on our own, not without community or family involvement. So becoming more systemic and therapeutic was kind of forced on us.

Rebecca: Was this a difficult shift to make?

Larry: Well, it was like learning to walk and falling down a lot–but we began to start working together to help our clients. The need to coordinate our efforts and come together seemed to be the only way to avoid sending double messages to children and their families. We had to work at being on the same page–as a team. There really wasn't anyone to guide us in this process, so we kind of learned by doing.

Theresa: But someone made the decision to start team work?

Larry: That's right–the new program director who came on in 1984. She had worked in a progressive child care agency in another state that was already using team work. She must have had a similar vision for The Children's Home and began the process of organizing around that concept.

As the team-centered approach began to take hold–or at least be experimented with–big changes began to occur.

Rebecca: Was there a huge turnover in staff?

Larry: Oh, huge! People were used to working independently and not having to explain why they were doing what they were doing or being called on the carpet for their actions.

Meribeth: As a direct care worker during that transition it was really hard. But good things came out of it too. In the past, for example, clinical supervision was not offered to direct care staff. Supervisors were mostly used when there were problems. Otherwise, you didn't meet regularly with any body. We just kind of did our own thing. When teams and formal supervisors were assigned, people were shaken up. You could no longer hide!

Larry: Some people were very upset with this shift–and upset with the Program Director for making these changes. But, really, it was necessary to have people in the upper levels of administration–including the Executive Director and the Board of Trustees–in support of such an important philosophical change.

Theresa: Can you talk a little bit about why the push for team work came first?

Rebecca: Well, I do think part of it was the new Program Director's vision along with support at the executive level. They recognized that learning how to work together and how to communicate with each other–the idea of team work–was imperative. At the same time, The Children's Home also began to be more therapeutically oriented.

Meribeth: That's right. We began paying more attention to programming issues–like family counseling, group work, individual issues. In the past that stuff happened on a sort of haphazard basis–it happened sometimes, but not in an intentional way. As team work began to take hold, we were able to attend to therapeutic needs more consistently.

Theresa: So in some sense, team and family-centered work began to emerge simultaneously–with maybe team work taking the lead.

Meribeth: Yes, I'd say that was the beginning of clinical work. The emphasis was on the individual or child at first–clinical work wasn't particularly family-centered but it was a start.

Larry: Being departmentalized and isolated hindered the clinical piece. Looking back, I realize we were re-creating what was happening in so many of the kids' homes–lack of communication between people, for example. It was like that story about the old yellow school bus Meribeth and I mentioned earlier–our old way of doing things kept breaking down half-way to our destination! Team work began to remedy this. But just putting us together and calling us teams didn't automatically make us teams.

Meribeth: That's right! We didn't really have a sense of who was supposed to be leading these teams, what people's roles were, or what a team ought to look like and be doing. It felt a bit like–"You will work together as a team–now go figure it out."

Larry: Also, because there was no clear hierarchy–at least that's my perception–informal power began to be exerted by those who were just charismatic or strong individuals and they would run the teams regardless of their positions. The teams would then fall into how that "personality" operated. But the creation of the Team Leader position helped address this problem.

Theresa: How so?

Larry: Team Leaders provided the clinical expertise because the position required a Master's degree in human services. They also were expected to supervise the direct care staff.

Meribeth: This addressed the lack of supervision and support for direct care staff. The agency also began to offer training to them and worked hard at helping to professionalize their positions–helping professionalize the field itself.

Larry: Even though we weren't doing family work as we know it today, we began talking about family work. We also began to experiment with more family-centered care through the development of an outreach program in another part of the state-reaching children and families without residential placement. So the plan was not necessarily overt that we were going to become more family-oriented. Really it was in the midst of doing teamwork that we began talking about working better with families and involving them more.

Theresa: And the Board of Trustees was supportive of this?

Larry: Yes, their support was important. Together we developed a new direction–or long-range plan–and began to operate differently.

Theresa: It's amazing how many of these things were happening concurrently. As we were learning to do teamwork, we were learning to be more systemic in our thinking and in what we were doing. This then translated to our work with families.

Larry: I also think focusing more on our work with families–helping children through helping their families–we realized the need to expand our range of services.

Theresa: If you could go back and do things over again, what do you think the organization could have done differently?

Meribeth: I think we've alluded to that some. Basically, as we went through the process of implementing team work, people really felt uprooted in many ways because of decisions that were made organizationally. They got rid of some old ways of doing things–even some positions. This created a great deal of insecurity among staff.

Larry: Yes, if I could go back and do it differently that's one of the things I'd pay more attention to–including people in the process more. People didn't really know what was happening–or at least the meaning of what was happening. It's like yanking the rug out of a room without moving any furniture–when you put the new rug down you *have* to move the furniture. People felt like they had no control. Teamwork is about empowering people and giving them control. But nobody felt like that in the beginning–except for a few people with vision and a passion for what was happening. The rest of the staff had no real explanation or sense of inclusion in the process.

Rebecca: Eventually, though, teams became empowered to make many more decisions than they had before. This was sometimes scary because it meant taking responsibility for mistakes as well as successes. People were credited *and* held accountable on a public level. We learned how to supervise more closely and help people get better at what they did–not just as individuals but as teams. That's also when we began to concentrate on relation ships within the agency. We worked hard at addressing issues around relationships that had been hidden–behavior that you sort of knew about but that never got dealt with or confronted. There was an expectation to deal with things more openly. And as we became less isolated, amazing resources emerged. We began to discover people's skills and strengths.

Larry: So, organizationally, we had to learn to apply clinical thinking to ourselves and to the organization itself–before we could really provide good services to our clients.

Rebecca: I think I personally went through a time when I realized that our behavior as professionals didn't always match the expectations we had of our clients. We had to be able to practice what we were preaching and not hide anymore.

Theresa: Did you also see a shift in power?

Larry: Yes. There was a shift in power from top administrators, who formerly made most decisions about placement and discharge, to those people working more directly with the children and families. Power became distributed more evenly. Input began to be sought from staff working directly with the kids.

Rebecca: So how did this shift toward shared decision-making occur?

Larry: I don't think it was internally driven at first–because The Children's Home had functioned the same way for a long time. As we talked about earlier, the type of children being referred began to change and the structure was no longer working. And then exciting things began to happen. As treatment teams were formed, they were taught how to communicate, share decisions, and interact with one another on behalf of their clients. Eventually, people at the administrative level saw the need to hold them selves to the same expectations being applied to treat ment teams. That's when the administrative team formed as well as teams related to program development and support. That was the next layer of teams created here. Aside from obvious core members, other people were invited to join these teams temporarily–as an experiment to see where they best fit.

Rebecca: Embracing team work across the entire agency was an important "experiment" that turned out to have lasting benefits. Before then, there were still remnants of departments. Well, we still have departments somewhat but they are gradually diminishing.

Larry: Sort of like the appendix. We still have it but we don't need it. We could have it removed but that would require surgery.

Meribeth: But evolution may take care of it–although slowly! Team retreats have helped us resolve some organizational issues more rapidly though. They also have helped people form a clearer picture of what being on a team requires and what benefits a well-functioning team brings.

Theresa: Which was the last team to be formed on campus?

Rebecca: The education team was the last to be created. There was some resistance about bringing together all the teachers and people connected to the school. I look back now and think, "Why?" I think it's ludicrous that we wouldn't have seen how obvious that need was. I guess hindsight is always much more informed. And I also think it's important to address in here what the resistance was about. In many ways it had to do with empowering people–some people gaining power or influence and other people feeling like they were losing it.

Theresa: There also probably was a fear that things might become too unwieldy in a team environment–especially with a group of people as large as the education team.

Rebecca: It's also important to weave in the whole issue of rela tionships because I think that's the other thing that's hap- pened through the process of developing team work. Ad- ministratively, we can see people and attend to them more easily. We have recognized that, if we attend to our staff and meet their needs, then certainly we are going to meet the needs of our clients much better.

Larry: So, in other words, in order to really be able to work with families, we had to start acting like a family–a healthy family. All the things you just described happen in a family. They communicate with each other, they have respect, they have relationships. When I first came here, staff did not socialize with each other. Trust level was extremely low.

Meribeth: And look what happens now! When staff leave here, they still have relationships with people on their teams. It seems to me this place makes a mark in people's lives.

Theresa: How do you think the administration has fit into all of this?

Larry: Well, I think recently the administrative team has made efforts to become more involved on a personal level. At one point they were overly involved in decision-making about clients then they backed away from this as they began to trust the team process more and the people that worked with clients on a daily basis. However, the pen- dulum may have swung too far–administration became somewhat underinvolved.

Rebecca: Even the most planned, positive shift can go too far if left to its own. But we're re-balancing and it's changing. There's a different level of involvement that's emerging at the administrative level–a healthy level of interest and investment.

Theresa.   Why do you think that happened?

Larry: Well, at one point, the administrative team never talked about the children except in the context of a crisis to be dealt with. But then we began a ritual at every meeting that included talking about our clients and their needs. I'd say every single member of the administrative team has had some child or family impact him or her in some way. They now follow some cases and inquire about them. Although we talk about the successes, we also talk about the hardships that led up to the successes. This has had an impact on people–and a huge impact on the Board of Trustees too. Board members now have a clearer picture of our clients changing needs.

Theresa: I also think a large part of the major change, at least in the last several years, happened because we had an Executive Director who was willing to let people do what they were good at doing and not second guess people or try to micro-manage what was going on. I'm not sure we could have undertaken a lot of the shifts we made if he had not been so supportive.

Larry: He also was eager to learn. He often had strong opinions and didn't always agree with what we were doing but he would still say, "Okay, I'll follow your lead." He was willing to trust the people he was working with.

Meribeth: He has been able to achieve that balance we talked about earlier–giving people space while also staying involved in strategic ways! That's a fine line–staying involved but not overly involved.

Theresa: And he meets every staff member.

Rebecca: Yes, he attends to relationships. That has helped create a strong sense of community. Paying attention to relationships is what helps build trust. And again, I really think teams were a tool to do that. Without them, it would have been much more difficult. Teams really helped us pay attention to each other.

Larry: Now I believe it's reached critical mass. Teamwork and family-centered care have taken on a life of their own and now are part of our agency culture. It's larger than the

> Executive Director or any subgroup of people. Our old ways have been absorbed and transformed, which wasn't a painless process. We had both growth and loss. But now we have a lot more freedom to be flexible and creative in the ways we serve people. We're learning how to be proactive and intentional with staff as well as clients.

Theresa: I like that we're still learning and changing as an agency. We haven't said, "Okay, this is it. We're done." Really, the process continues to unfold. And that's exciting.

The four staff dialoguing in this article are members of the Consultation and Training Team at The Children's Home, Inc. in Winston-Salem, North Carolina. This team has been providing consultation and training since 1992 to organizations in the residential field. The Consultation and Training Team offers specific curriculum designed to promote team development and family-centered practice.

BIOGRAPHICAL NOTES

Rebecca S. Barboff, MS, LMFT. Current position: Program Director, 11 years at The Children's Home, Inc. Previous positions include: Child Care Worker, Social Worker, Cottage Life Coordinator, and Program Manager.

M. Theresa Palmer, MSW. Current position: Family Counselor for Early Intervention and Prevention, 6 years at The Children's Home, Inc. Previous positions include: Resident Counselor and Team Leader.

Meribeth Robinson, MS. Current position: Assistant Program Director, 14 years at The Children's Home, Inc. Previous positions include: Child Care Worker, Lead Worker, and Team Leader.

Larry B. Sharpe, CCSW, AAMFT Approved Supervisor. Current position: Director of Family Services and Training, 16 years at The Children's Home, Inc. Previous positions include: House Parent, Social Worker, Outreach Coordinator, and Program Director.

"Progress"

That first week he asked
what make of car I drove,
adding with some impertinence,
"I thought any doctor
worth his salt, drove
a long, black Cadillac."

The second week he volunteered,
"You've got the right build
for a Cadillac," pointing
to my annual winter paunch,
now petitioning to become
perennial, by hanging 'round
on the verge of summer.

Smart-alec kid, I thought.

Come fall he had conceded,
somewhat gratuitously
it seemed to me, but
nevertheless, kind of him,
that my build more nearly
matched the geriatric Chevy
pick-up that I drove.

It is gratifying to note
that he's no longer
such a smart-alec kid,

[Haworth co-indexing entry note]: "Progress." Powers, Douglas. Co-published simultaneously in *Residential Treatment for Children & Youth* (The Haworth Press, Inc.) Vol. 17, No. 3, 2000, pp. 77-78; and: *Family-Centered Services in Residential Treatment: New Approaches for Group Care* (ed: John Y. Powell) The Haworth Press, Inc., 2000, pp. 77-78. Single or multiple copies of this article are available for a fee from The Haworth Document Delivery Service [1-800-342-9678, 9:00 a.m. - 5:00 p.m. (EST). E-mail address: getinfo@haworthpressinc.com].

the way he used to be;
and to know that he can
learn something. . . anything
if one can muster patience.

Douglas Powers, MD

Questioning the Continuum of Care: Toward a Reconceptualization of Child Welfare Services

Earl N. Stuck, Jr.
Richard W. Small
Frank Ainsworth

SUMMARY. The notion of a "continuum of care" and the associated idea of residential care and treatment programs for children and youth as "last resort" interventions are endemic in the child welfare literature (Whittaker, 1979; Beker, 1981). The purpose of this paper is to question the utility of both of these notions. Indeed, it will be argued that the construct of a continuum of care as it plays out in practice is fundamentally problematic, inhibiting the use of appropriately intensive interventions even when they are in the best interests of children and families, and inhibiting rather than promoting family reunification in many complex cases. *[Article copies available for a fee from The Haworth Document Delivery Service: 1-800-342-9678. E-mail address: getinfo@haworthpressinc.com <Website: http://www.haworthpressinc.com>]*

KEYWORDS. Reconceptualization of a continuum of care, integrated array of child and family services, residential care as a family support service

A version of this paper was first presented at the 1995 Child Welfare League of America annual conference in Washington, DC. Comments from many of our colleagues shaped this final version. Special thanks to Cyndi Smith, and to Jake Terpstra of the U.S. Children's Bureau for his especially detailed and helpful suggestions.

The authors may be written at Walker Trieschman Center, 300 Congress Street, Suite 305, Quincey, MA 02169.

[Haworth co-indexing entry note]: "Questioning the Continuum of Care: Toward a Reconceptualization of Child Welfare Services." Stuck, Earl N. Jr., Richard W. Small, and Frank Ainsworth. Co-published simultaneously in *Residential Treatment for Children & Youth* (The Haworth Press, Inc.) Vol. 17, No. 3, 2000, pp. 79-92; and: *Family-Centered Services in Residential Treatment: New Approaches for Group Care* (ed: John Y. Powell) The Haworth Press, Inc., 2000, pp. 79-92. Single or multiple copies of this article are available for a fee from The Haworth Document Delivery Service [1-800-342-9678, 9:00 a.m. - 5:00 p.m. (EST). E-mail address: getinfo@haworthpressinc.com].

EMERGENCE OF THE CONTINUUM OF CARE
AS A METAPHOR FOR SERVICE DELIVERY

During the past century, the field of children's services has become highly diversified, yet it did not start out that way. For most of this nation's history, there were few recognized options for children. Orphanages, apprenticeships, reform schools, alms houses, and informal kinship care largely represented the main components of a loose system of child welfare. These generally reflected a viewpoint that society's responsibilities to children were limited to the fairly basic provision of care and the correction of antisocial behavior. Managed primarily by church communities, the system of care as well as its sources of funding were largely voluntary and parochial for most of the first two centuries of this nation's history (Bremer, 1971).

The last half century has witnessed the proliferation of a vast array of services to meet the many needs of children and their families. Each in turn represented an innovation, a new way of looking at children in response to their changing needs, as well as recognition of the advances in the technology of care. Alms houses and orphanages gave way to family foster care, adoption and enlightened schools for the reform of wayward youth.

As the life expectancy of the citizenry increased, and the waves of immigration declined throughout the Great Depression, so also did the number of true orphans. Society began to recognize that even when children had parents, they sometimes did not receive adequate care in safe surroundings. They often fared poorly, both socially and educationally. The effects of parental abuse and neglect were increasingly documented. There was an acknowledged need for new interventions to provide both for basic needs as well as remedial and therapeutic supports. Children who needed basic care were usually referred temporarily to relatives or family foster care. Orphanages struggled to adapt to the increasingly troubled children who could not be maintained in family settings. Some of these closed, while others diversified and developed sophisticated approaches to the treatment of a range of social, behavioral and emotional disturbances. Today's residential treatment centers in their many forms are the outgrowth of this evolutionary change.

In the latter half of this century, child welfare services became more complex and sophisticated, and more expensive. The major sources of support for these programs gradually shifted from the churches and other private groups and individuals, to the public sector. Government saw its significant interest in both the protection of children, and in the promotion of quality services to help overcome the effects of past abuse and neglect. The recognition of society's responsibility to act "in the best interest of the child" resulted in the proliferation of a great variety of out-of-home care services during the 60's and 70's. At the same time, partly in recognition of the cost, and partly due to the prevailing cultural belief that children are best raised in their families, many other services focused on providing the support necessary to maintain children in their homes, and when removed, to reunify families or find other permanent families. Home-based family services, day treatment, child day care, and a variety of community-based family services developed with the goal of strengthening the capacity of families to care for their own children safely.

What the evolving system developed was a tremendous variety of care and service options. What the system did not have was coordination, nor a generally accepted way of determining when, where, and under what conditions these services should be provided. By the mid 1970s, at a time when nearly one half million children were in the child welfare system, having been determined to have been abused and/or neglected, there was a need to provide order to decisions that had great ramifications for the shape and substance of the service system, as well as the overall cost of such a system to the public. In 1980, with the passage of the Adoption Assistance and Child Welfare Act (P.L. 96272), a system was created that has been in place to this day. The new law determined that no child would be removed from a home unless he or she was shown to be at imminent risk of harm and that the authorities must make "reasonable efforts" to assure safety and maintain the child in the home wherever possible. If the child was removed, the subsequent placement needed to be in the "least restrictive" (originally intended to mean closest to home) setting available that could meet the child's and family's needs. Use of more restrictive and intensive interventions, such as residential treatment, could only be made when less intensive interventions were judged to be ineffective. At all times, "reasonable efforts" to prevent placement and to reunify families were required by law.

The 1980 legislation is the foundation of the "continuum of care" as a case management blueprint governing most decisions in child welfare today. The underlying beliefs of the continuum include:

- Children are to be raised in the home unless there can be proven risk to safety.
- The use of more restrictive interventions, especially out-of-home care, carry the inherent risk of harm to the child through broken family connections and institutionalization.
- Therefore, services should be considered for children and families in a linear, step-wise fashion, from least to most restrictive, as this approach is most likely to keep families together.
- Placement into group care should only be utilized as a last resort.

These underlying beliefs have attracted widespread support as they are consistent with and influenced by the ideologies of normalization, deinstitutionalization, mainstreaming, minimal intervention and diversion that have powerfully influenced all of human services for the last twenty-five years (Fulcher and Ainsworth, 1994). The idea that the least intensive or intrusive services should always be used first has also found powerful support from fiscal decision makers allied to monetarist economic policies (Culpitt, 1992), as a key rationalization for reducing public funding for human services. Finally, ideology aside, the notion of a linear, prescriptive continuum has appeal for very practical reasons. Over the past two decades, the child welfare system has grown dramatically. Case decisions have increasingly been made by social service departments experiencing the stress of rising client caseloads due to court orders for care and the impact of mandated reporting (Hutchison, 1993), high turnover and large number of new workers cycling through the system, and the simultaneous pressure of budget cutting and increasing public skepticism of social programs. The continuum notion allows for patterned, politically viable case management decisions by even the most inexperienced workers.

PROBLEMS WITH THE CONTINUUM AS A PRACTICE BLUEPRINT

Conceptually, while the continuum of care is based on the principle that the least restrictive of *appropriate* alternatives be utilized, only sporadic guidelines exist to assure that children consistently receive individualized appropriate care. The result has been a linear model for care that, in implementation, creates serious practical problems for both care providers and the children and families they serve. In a real sense, the continuum has become a one-way street children and families must travel until they reach the point where the system can meet their needs at that time or until diversion of the child client into mental health or youth corrections takes the pressure off the system all together. The road leads always toward the more intensive services, but offers few opportunities to double back, pull off, or check the road map without having to start the helping process all over again. Specifically, the continuum as a guideline for practice trades the ease of patterned decisions for the accuracy of decisions based upon individual assessment of the child's and family's strengths and needs.

In a rather typical example of how the continuum defines intervention, a child is identified as being at risk of abuse. If the child welfare system has the resources, efforts are made to strengthen the home and to assist the parents to successfully raise the child. Too often, the problems are not recognized early enough to prevent harm, but only after real harm has occurred. Since the system's first response is usually with preventative services, the response may already be one click too late, a pattern which can come to be a feature of the system throughout.

Perhaps, however, if further abuse or neglect occurs, and also the child begins to display behavioral and emotional problems, at some relatively arbitrary point the decision is made to provide family preservation services. As distinguished from ongoing family support, these services are intensive, but mostly time limited. After a relatively brief try, these services are either assessed to have worked, in which case the family is usually effectively dropped from the case load with little further support, or continued abuse is identified, in which case the child is removed and placed in temporary foster care. From this point on, the family, which may now be labeled as "unworkable" or "resistant," moves increasingly further out of the picture. Because the child is not only the victim of abuse, but also may be acting out at escalating levels, the first foster home placement fails, beginning a trail of repeated attempts to "find the right match."

At some point, the frustrated worker has established a significant enough resume of failure for this client to present the case for residential group treatment. The child's biological family, which has ceased to be the primary focus of service many stops ago, may now be described in the record as "not identifiable." The child is disconnected, yet reunification remains the system's formal goal. The residential center works with the child in a vacuum, receiving (or, to be fair, perhaps choosing to hear) the dual messages from the placing agency to keep the stay brief, but leave the family to us. If the child does well, and returns home, transitional and aftercare services are too often unavailable. The family, having been largely left out of the process, has little support and few new skills with which to cope. Too often the scenario leading to placement begins again. To compound the problem, the child usually is not returned to the place where she/he last received care, eliminating the chance to build on previous interventions helpful to the child and family.

FUNDAMENTAL CONCEPTUAL FLAWS

We believe the helping process can and does play out as in the above example because of some very fundamental flaws in the concept of continuum.

There Are Logical Inconsistencies in the "Least Restrictive" Standard

The "least restrictive" standard in the 1980 Adoption Assistance and Child Welfare Act is at the conceptual heart of the continuum of care. Unfortunately, as implemented, in real-life systems, it can also be the biggest logical inconsistency. "Least restrictive," like its "least intrusive" counterpart in medicine is only important as a guide to *whether* and *when* to intervene, not to decide *how*. The surgeon should not pick up a scalpel until he is certain that less intrusive measures are unlikely to work. However, once this decision is made, he cuts as deeply as his assessment of the patient's *individual case* warrants. While "least restrictive" may be a fair indicator of when the child welfare system should intervene in a family, it cannot be the primary rule governing the nature of the intervention. Yet in child welfare practice, this is very often exactly the case. The result is an incremental approach to practice intervention wherein individual assessments are overridden by the systemic bias to begin with step-down helping options.

Progress Along the Continuum Advances by Failure

An approach that requires that the least intensive interventions should always be used first results in a system with case management decisions driven by failure. As in the example above, family-based foster care is the intervention of choice for a child entering out-of-home care for the first time, as it is the least intensive, least costly option. Most of the time, only if family foster care fails, usually repeatedly, is more intensive intervention given consideration. This is in spite of evidence that the number of placements a child experiences has a negative impact on a child's development, and heavily influences the child's condition at the point of exit from care (Fanshel, Finch and Grundy, 1990). The presumption of the continuum in practice is that one uses an intervention not only until it does not work, but until one can prove that it cannot work. While this is arguable proof against the use of more restrictive (and expensive) services too early, it also increases the chance they will be used too late.

"Progress by Failure" Biases the System Towards Crisis and Blame

Movement from one stop along the continuum to another only after certified failure creates a negatively-biased system adept at recognizing risk, weakness and pathology far more effectively than strengths in individuals and families. The system tends to mobilize only around problems, with case decisions too often made in response to crisis. For those clients who remain in the system over time and make the long journey from least to most restrictive services, repeated failure can mean blame and alienation. Helpers and families increasingly relate not through partnership, but through corrective action plans demanding compliance. Connections between children and biological families are eroded or broken, only to find that when exit from the system is imminent, the resources and motivation needed to make the reunification plan work are missing. Likewise, the "trial by fire" process of reaching the proper level of care tends to destroy other resources along the way. In particular, experience has given us many examples of highly motivated, caring foster parents who eventually burned out because they were unable to cope with very troubled children, well after it should have been evident that more intensive interventions were warranted. The bottom line is progress by failure for child, family, and helpers alike, with each party tending to blame the other at every new crisis point.

Realistic Family Reunification Is Compromised

The hierarchy of least intensive helping services as "good for families" and most intensive helping services as "bad for families" widely believed imposed on the continuum by the 1980 legislation (though not in fact, spelled out in P.L. 96272 as written), in part based on the ideological position that truly functional families should raise their children with little or no outside support, also leads to an overly rigid definition of family reunification. Within this hierarchy, if incremental, time-limited services fail to prevent placement, complete separation of child and family usually results. At the other end of the continuum, work toward reunification of children in out-of-home care is seen as fully successful only if it is full-time reunification, the child returning home with minimal family support. In fact, the above premises are far too simplistic. Real-life practice suggests that family reunification should be defined more broadly as helping each child and family achieve and maintain, at any given time, the optimal level of reconnection from full reentry into the family system to other forms of contact such as visiting or shared care, that affirm the child's membership in the family (Warsh, Maluccio and Pine, 1994, p. 3). From this point of view, optimum family connections are compromised by a hierarchical continuum of intervention and practice methods within which reunification is a "pass-fail" event.

Boundaries Between Services Are Overly Rigid

One of the most perplexing problems with the continuum concept is that it leads to case management as a series of digital decisions, i.e., either family preservation or out-of-home care; either reunification or termination of parental rights, etc. This means there is little possibility to mix and use various services in combination. The *sequential* delivery philosophy interferes with the possibility that *simultaneous* interventions may be appropriate. The fact that a child has been removed from home because a family-focused intervention appears not to have worked should not mean that intensive family work ceases, quite to the contrary in many cases.

A side effect of overly rigid boundaries is competition among services in the continuum, with the "good" (i.e., less restrictive) services defining their value in terms of preventing the "bad" (i.e., more intensive) services. Residential group care, for instance, is seen as the failure outcome of family preservation, strongly inhibiting the possibilities of integration. The capacity of a range of services to support a common goal is compromised by the competition both for resources and the political high ground of being the "correct" service for children.

BEYOND THE CONTINUUM:
TOWARD A CARE MANAGEMENT SERVICE SYSTEM

Notwithstanding the above critique, it is important to acknowledge that for many families needing services of limited intensity and duration, the continuum of care and least restrictive notion helped to humanize child welfare services over the last 20 years. Foster care services have expanded and now serve a range of children who previously might have been placed in residential facilities. Treatment facilities for children and young people are no longer segregated, isolated institutions, distanced from the surrounding community, where children only have contact with staff and other residents.

Child care institutions, consisting of large congregate living units surrounded by an extensive although socially restrictive campus, have in the main given way to smaller, more culturally normative facilities. No longer isolated, many of these facilities have developed innovative, community based group care options. In addition, minor offenders are no longer placed for extended periods in training schools where the delinquent subculture tended to oppose reform attempts. Diversionary programs now try to keep legal intervention low key and to a sensible minimum.

But the ultimate question remains: is the incremental, implicitly hierarchical approach to service at the core of the continuum of care appropriate to the high risk children and families increasingly flooding the child welfare system? We think the answer is clearly no. Yet giving up the linear rigidity in the continuum notion as a blueprint for case management does not have to mean giving up family preservation or fiscal responsibility as cornerstone values. Indeed, our colleagues in health care have already learned that successful managed care with the high risk, even chronically ill populations is possible, but it is best understood as a process of "illness management," in which the emphasis is not on the success or failure of particular interventions but on the overall status of a person over the course of a whole lifetime. Within this model, the most aggressive interventions are not necessarily avoided or implemented as a last resort, but justified at various points in time as ultimately supportive of long-term stabilization based on the individual needs of the patient and his family. While we emphatically do not intend to equate the needs of children and families in the child welfare system with illness or disease, we nevertheless believe that this way of thinking about services to the most vulnerable families may have great value for child welfare as an alternative to current formulations of the continuum of care. Taking a "care management" approach to the longest term, highest risk clients in the system allows an approach to service implementation which would:

- acknowledge that some children and families will require services at various levels of intensity over time, and that this may be a decidedly nonlinear process. From this perspective, the challenge becomes to provide appropriate (including appropriately limited) interventions at various points in time; to design each intervention as part of a continuous strategy of family stabilization so that past, present, and future interventions shape each other; and to manage helping resources for each family over time rather than seek quick-fix solutions;
- retain the emphasis on family empowerment and family connections at all levels of service, but recognize that optimum connections may not mean that every parent and child lives together full-time, or over the entire minority of the child without ongoing support;
- put a premium on continuous, coordinated assessment where the operative question is not where does the child and family fit into the system, but rather how do services in the system best fit the child and family needs at the time;
- put an equal premium on care and support to families *after* the course of intensive services, as a way of preventing costly future interventions as much as possible emphasize the choice of least restrictive (and costly) *appropriate* service for children and families, investing in intensive interventions at the outset and throughout the course of care if assessment dictates this is the best bet for dealing with trauma and/or for keeping families together over the long haul
- blend services so there are step-up and step-down options at all levels of intervention, and in particular so that the rigid boundaries between home-based and out-of-home services are eliminated;
- develop outcomes, including cost-benefit measures, not limited solely to discrete services but to long-range family stabilization and the real cost of services across time.

At the very least, taking this care management approach allows us to transform the continuum into a more integrated array of child and family services (see Figure 1). Especially noteworthy here is that, once and for all, the characterization of residential group care as a "last resort"/failure outcome is replaced with a view of residential options in support of families at all levels of the service system. As is clear from Figure 2, this greatly expands the potential range of creative uses of residential services. Of course, the challenge for those of us within the field of group care will be to retool significantly how, when, and where group care services get delivered.

We do not expect either the critique or the revision of the continuum in this paper to go unchallenged. However, we do expect this concep-

FIGURE 1. Child and Family Services

Continuum of Care

–Services used up one at a time
–Progress through failure in other systems
–Least intensive vs. most appropriate
–Residential care as last resort
–Least intensive equated with family supportive

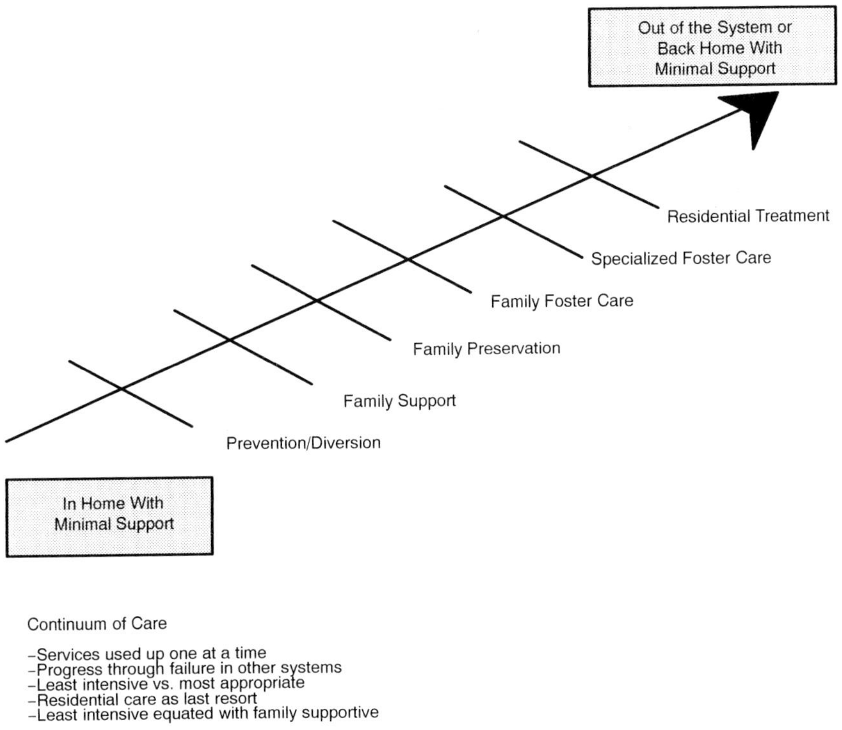

FIGURE 2. Community Services in Support of Children and Families

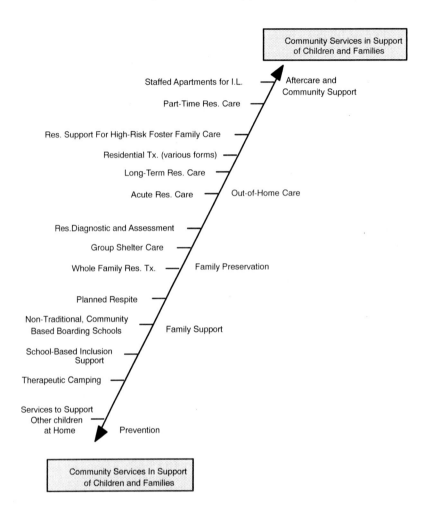

Case Management Service Array

–Residential care as support for families and other services, not last resort/failure outcome.
–Services integrated rather than sequential. Some children move both in and out of high intensity services over time
–Broad definition of family reunification
–Clients enter the system at various points based on individual assessment

tion of care management within a flexible array of services supporting a wide-range of reunification options, or something like it, will shape the political and economic future of child welfare services for years to come. We invite response from our colleagues.

REFERENCES

Ainsworth, F. and Fulcher, L.C. (1994). *Ideology and the abandonment of child welfare*. Manuscript submitted for publication.

Atherton, C. (1969). The social assignment of social work. *Social Services Review,* 43, 3, 421-429.

Beker, J. (1981). New roles for group care centers. In F. Ainsworth and L.C. Fulcher. *Group care for children: concept and issue.* London: Tavistock Publications.

Bremer, R.H. (Ed.) (1971). Children and youth in America: Volume I and 11. Cambridge, MA: Harvard University Press.

Culpitt, l. (1992). *Welfare and citizenship: beyond the crisis of the welfare state.* London, Sage Publications.

Fanshel, D., Finch, S.J. and Grundy, J.F. (1990). *Foster children in life course perspective.* New York, NY: Columbia University Press.

Hutchison, E.D. (1993). Mandatory reporting laws: child protection case findings gone awry? *Social Work,* 38, 1, 56-63.

Warsh, R. Maluccio, A.N. and Pine, B. (1994) (Eds.) *Together again. Family reunification in foster care.* Washington, DC: Child Welfare League of America.

Whittaker, J.K. (1979). *Caring for troubled children.* San Francisco, CA: Jossey-Bass.

BIOGRAPHICAL NOTES

Earl Stuck, Jr., is a well-known teacher and lecturer on subjects such as administration, group care, juvenile justice and youth issues, and working with families of children and youth in out-of-home care. Mr. Stuck serves as Associate Director for the Child Welfare League of America's National Center for Consultation and Professional Development.

Richard Small, Ph.D., has served as the Executive Director of the Walker Home and School since 1985. Mr. Small is an author, educator, and consultant to child welfare programs around the world. He also served as Executive Director of the Massachusetts Governor's advisory Committee on Child and the Family. He served as a consultant and primary writer for the Carolinas Project.

Frank Ainsworth holds an academic position at Edith Cowan University in Perth, Western Australia. He has also held similar positions in Britain and the US. He has a longstanding interest in child and youth care issues, especially residential practice. Mr. Ainsworth is well known internationally through his extensive publications on these topics.

Space Talk

Roy, a scruffy kid of ten
Moved in with worn suitcase,
While all the others stood
Eying him up and down.

"I wish Jim was still here;
And I wish he'd write to us,"
A boy in back said wistfully,
"I think I liked him better."

"Roy's taking Jimbo's place,"
The counselor tried a smile.
"You'll all like Roy, too,
After he's been here awhile."

Roy shrugged practiced shoulders:
"I've never taken anyone's place.
And if this is like all the others
Just consider it a borrowed space."

Douglas Powers, MD

[Haworth co-indexing entry note]: "Space Talk." Powers, Douglas. Co-published simultaneously in *Residential Treatment for Children & Youth* (The Haworth Press, Inc.) Vol. 17, No. 3, 2000, p. 93; and: *Family-Centered Services in Residential Treatment: New Approaches for Group Care* (ed: John Y. Powell) The Haworth Press, Inc., 2000, p. 93. Single or multiple copies of this article are available for a fee from The Haworth Document Delivery Service [1-800-342-9678, 9:00 a.m. - 5:00 p.m. (EST). E-mail address: getinfo@haworthpressinc.com].

Looking Back to See Ahead

James M. Campbell, MS

My wife, who is a professor of reading, tells me that most of what we read and most of the conversations in which we engage, amount to little more than stories. We use stories to describe the world around us, events we participate in, interactions in which we engage, and to tell others who we are.

This conference is entitled *Fresh Thinking About Group Care for Children*. For us to begin to think about ideas, it often helps to look to the past as prelude. So bear with me because I am going to tell you some stories which I hope will capture a small historical era when I was a recipient of group care for children.

I believe that two caveats are in order before I begin. First, I am mindful that two fellow alumni from Barium Springs Orphanage during my stay there are in the audience. For me to say disrespectful things about our home would probable be tantamount to one of you "talking bad" about your mother. But guys, these are my memories. I promise you that I will not engage in revisionist history by trying to hold anyone account-

Professor Campbell's address was delivered at a 1997 East Carolina University Symposium, "Fresh Thinking About Group Care for Children." He grew up at Barium Springs Home for Children in North Carolina, and he reflected upon his experiences there with a view of what aspects of group care might be retained from the past and what should be changed or added for today's children.

It should be noted that Barium Springs Home for Children is a now a modern, progressive child care agency that provides multiple services for children and their families.

The author may be written at the School of Social Work and Criminal Justice Studies, East Carolina University, Greenville, NC 27858.

[Haworth co-indexing entry note]: "Looking Back to See Ahead." Campbell, James M. Co-published simultaneously in *Residential Treatment for Children & Youth* (The Haworth Press, Inc.) Vol. 17, No. 3, 2000, pp. 95-102; and: *Family-Centered Services in Residential Treatment: New Approaches for Group Care* (ed: John Y. Powell) The Haworth Press, Inc., 2000, pp. 95-102. Single or multiple copies of this article are available for a fee from The Haworth Document Delivery Service [1-800-342-9678, 9:00 a.m. - 5:00 p.m. (EST). E-mail address: getinfo@haworthpressinc.com].

able for knowledge, beliefs, philosophies, or practices of today. I believe that most of my care givers did the best they could with their knowledge, skills and abilities and the prevailing practices of that day.

The second caveat is that my expertise is in criminal justice, not in social welfare or child care. My remarks are those of one who has "been there, done that," and as an older observer of the social landscape. If I say anything that contradicts child welfare practice and philosophy please ignore what I say and listen to the experts.

I graduated from Barium Springs High School in May of 1956. This school was located on the grounds of the Presbyterian Orphans Home at Barium Springs, North Carolina. At the time of my graduation I was 17 years old and had been a resident of that orphanage for 15 years. Because I had no skills and no place to go, and since there was a compulsory military draft anyway, I decided to enlist in the Air Force.

Let me digress here for a moment. Try to imagine, if you will, where you were and how you processed the world when you were only seventeen. Now try to imagine yourself at that age with no safety net beneath you, no home to go to, no job, no skills except that of farm laborer, no older and wiser parent or adult advisor to whom you could turn, and the understanding that as of graduation day you were expected to leave the only home you had known since you were three.

That was me at age seventeen. And at the end of this first difficult day of military service, I was sitting on my footlocker in Texas, looking around and surveying the seventy or so other young men with whom I would be sharing the next two months of basic training.

Around me I heard the occasional whisper (since we were forbidden to talk out loud) about maybe this was all a mistake, another whisper that "I sure would like to be eating mama's cooking," and several sniffles of young men desperately trying to hold back the tears and to deal with the first pangs of homesickness.

As I witnessed these scenes being enacted all around me I suddenly broke out in a huge grin. It suddenly dawned on me that I was home! Yes, I was with strangers and my drill instructor cursed and screamed at me and required me to stand in rigid positions, salute and march everywhere I went. But I was home. Even though everything around me was new, I recognized it all. I was in a dormitory (although they called it a barracks), there was order, routine and discipline. And wonder of all wonders they gave me snappy uniforms and paid me the princely sum of $75.00 a month, more money than I had ever seen.

Over the years I have come to believe that I was probably dealing for the first time with the results of long term institutionalization. And it has taken me most of my adult life to completely rid myself of it. In fact, vestiges of it still remain. For example, my wife kindly and graciously has come to realize that I really am not comfortable spending the night in someone else's home. You must remember that for the first twenty one years of my life I had little or no knowledge of a private dwelling house and that my life was connected to barracks and dormitories.

In the past several years there has been an interest in and probably a small movement toward the notion of "revisiting" the orphanage. Much of this is probably fueled by people of my age who, after being reared in an orphanage, and having enjoyed a successful life, begin to call for a return to the concept of the orphanage that they knew. It seems that they forget that time, practices, and law have changed dramatically the home they remembered.

There are two reasons why I believe that the slice of Americana we call the orphanage is no longer with us and why, in my opinion, it will never return–as we knew it. The first of these reasons concerns the failure of the institution as panacea and the second is the individual rights revolution of the 1960's and 70's.

THE FAILURE OF THE INSTITUTION AS PANACEA

David Rothman, in his book *The Discovery of the Asylum* maintains that early in the nineteenth century (around 1830's) there emerged the idea in America that we could cure many of our social ills with the creation of the institution. The proponents of institutions looked around them and saw poverty, mental illness, the blind, criminal offenders, juvenile delinquency, and orphans. These social reformers believed that many of the unfortunate persons finding themselves in these conditions were there due to the contagion or corruption in the community and the family. Therefore, if they could only build institutions in the rural, uncontaminated places of America, and relocate the unfortunate victims of these social ills to these institutions, then with the inculcation of religious values, education, discipline, and hard work these problems could be cured. And if there was success then these institutions could serve as models of how to treat social problems and models for the larger society to follow and, in effect, would cure all of these problems. So the institution became the panacea for many social ills.

Unfortunately, Rothman says, during the nineteenth century, one could go from a prison to a mental hospital to a poor house to an orphanage and not notice a dime's worth of difference. The buildings were the same, the internal processes were the same, and the vocabulary was the same. Later when I begin to speak about my experiences there I will call the women responsible for me "matrons." I realize the politically correct name today would be "housemother," or "house parent," however, it was the name used in my day. Notice also, that at the same time, female guards in prisons, jails, mental hospitals and other institutions were called matrons.

When you look around at many state and private institutions today, traces and vestiges of this "brick and mortar" institutional mentality can still be observed. And in some of our cities in North Carolina one can see that over time the city has grown and has swallowed up the once rural characteristic of the institution, but the large buildings still remain; for example Central Prison and Dorethea Dix Mental Hospital in Raleigh.

Sometime around the turn of the century this institutional philosophy began to change but it would take until the legal rights revolution of the 1960's and 70's to really propel the change. Maybe economic times were better and we just didn't need the orphanage any longer, or maybe we began to realize that the institution was not necessarily the answer to all of our social problems. Maybe it was new knowledge in psychology, sociology, social work, medicine, and other physical and social sciences that proposed other responses to these problems.

I was the ninth child of a blue-collar mill worker and his wife. I was born near the end of what is now called the Great Depression of the 1930's. All around me, as well as throughout the South, although I did not know it until I was an adult, there was poverty everywhere. I was twelve months old when my father died, and 18 months old when my mother died. There was an attempt by my older siblings and an elderly grandmother to keep the family together. But after a year of desperately trying, a plea was made by someone in our behalf to the Presbyterian Home for Children at Barium Springs, North Carolina.

After the caseworker completed her investigation it was decided that the five youngest children, ranging from ages 12 to 3, were to be institutionalized. I have no recollection of mother or father, nor do I remember going to the orphanage. To this day all that I remember of my childhood was my life at Barium Springs. As a side note, my family represented only a small fraction of the 300 or so children at

Barium Springs who were true orphans. Most of the children there were from single parent homes.

In keeping with the prevailing philosophy of that day, all children in the orphanage were segregated by age and sex. Thus, I never was able to stay with or be raised around any of my siblings who accompanied me there. This has resulted in a lifelong quasi-alienation from my siblings, and I am closer to some of the boys I was raised with than my own family.

In the central dining hall seating arrangements were by "cottages." My sister tells me that on the day of our arrival she heard me crying at my table and the matron in charge of me saying that if I did not stop crying I would get no food. She left her table, went over to mine, picked me up and took me to her table and held and fed me. Of course, this was a serious breach of regulations, and she was punished for it.

The "cottages" we were assigned to were not cottages, but rather, were massive structures. And one moved from one cottage to another as he/she advanced in age. With the changes to different cottages came different degrees of freedom and responsibility. So that by the time I was in the sixth grade, I was rising at about 5:00 a.m. and, with other boys my age, milking about 40 milk cows, feeding calves, tending to steers, and then jointly cleaning the milking barn. Then we went to breakfast and later to school. After school, this work responsibility was repeated.

On through high school we were assigned to work in apple and peach orchards, work on produce farms and combining grain and gathering in hay. Some of the boys were assigned to work in the orphanage printing shop, the shoe shop, the carpenter shop, and the plumbing shop.

Girls were assigned to "women's work" such as working in the laundry, shelling lima beans, snapping green beans, and several were assigned to assist the matrons with their young charges in the various cottages. As you can imagine, the work ethic was alive and well at Barium Springs. They probably believed most vociferously that "an idle hand is the devil's workshop." This work ethic, however, did not occur in a vacuum. All around us in rural and urban North Carolina and in this nation, young boys and girls were required to work and learned the important lesson that honest labor is good for the body as well as the soul.

The daily routine we experienced, especially for the younger children, was very prescribed. We marched in columns of two to school, we were called to the dining hall by a tower bell, allowed to enter the dining hall by the person in charge there ringing a hand bell, and then a call for silence for the blessing of the meal by a smaller tap bell, and after the allotted time for the meal, a bell announced that we were to leave the dining hall.

The orphanage had its own school, with most of the teachers who were single living in apartments or rooms provided by the orphanage. Most of our teachers not only supervised us in the classroom, but on the campus, in the dining hall, and anywhere else they would encounter us.

And, of course, there was religious instruction. We were required to attend Sunday school, Sunday morning worship service, and youth group meetings on Sunday nights. We were required to attend Wednesday night prayer service and occasionally to attend revival services. Religious instruction carried over into the classroom as well, so that every boy and girl there were required to take a course in the Old Testament during the tenth grade, and the New Testament in the twelfth. And one of the requirements for successful completion of this course was that everyone had to preach a sermon, ten minutes long, and could not use a watch in the process.

Once again, if this religious instruction was forced upon some of us and lovingly sought after by others, then this was also the condition of young men and women in the larger community so that we were not alone.

What I am describing for you, as I remember it, was a total institution. All employees of Barium Springs from the superintendent to the supervisors at the orchards, dairy, and the farm, to our matrons and their male counterparts, everyone, had a say in our development, our deportment, our responsibility for being on time and doing what we were supposed to be doing or else. And corporal punishment could and was inflicted by all of these people for serious offenders of the rules. For the most part, and with only one or two minor exceptions, it is an experience that I will always treasure. It gave me a warm and secure place where I was never in fear of being shunted from one home to another or being thrown into the streets. There was abundant food. There was instilled in me the value of hard work. I received what I consider to be, for that time and place, an excellent education. And I was given religious instruction which helped shape my morals.

THE INDIVIDUAL RIGHTS REVOLUTION

All through the 1960's and 1970's the United States Supreme Court began, through its rulings, to interpret the Constitution to mean that individuals in America, including those in institutions, had a certain body of rights which heretofore had been denied to them. For example, in the late nineteenth century, the Supreme Court in the case of *Ruffin v. Commonwealth* ruled that a prisoner being held in a state penitentiary was a "slave of the state" and was entitled to only those things or rights granted to him by a benevolent state. This all began to change in the mid-twentieth century when the Supreme Court began to do what individual states up to that time had failed to do. It began to say that when people were institutionalized that it must be done with due process of law, and that while they were institutionalized that there were a significant body of rights attendant to the conditions of that confinement.

The court also began to rule, as in the landmark case of *In Re Gault* concerning the rights of juvenile offenders in the adjudicatory process, that sometimes the best intentions of the helping professions were not good enough. That sometimes bad things happened to children in the name of doing good. Thus, we began to see the erosion, if not the complete removal, of the concept of "benevolent purpose" which had guided human service providers for so many years.

As a result of many of these Supreme Court rulings, we began to empty out our mental hospitals, our juvenile training schools (in Massachusetts they were closed down). We began to develop more humane treatments of criminal offenders and today the beat goes on to ensure that elderly and disadvantaged persons are not mistreated in institutions.

If we tried to superimpose the orphanage in which I was raised in today's society here is what I believe we would face. Racially segregated facilities would not be tolerated, especially if tax funds were used to support it. Religious instruction would probable cease or be severely curtailed. Corporal punishment would cease, especially that which would be considered excessive or abusive. I can recall liberal use of the razor strop, "peachtree tea," belts, milking machine hoses, and of course the hand and the foot.

Most work requirements would probably be in violation of federal and state law. I can remember, at ages twelve to sixteen, cutting silage corn with a machete with no protective gear on my legs. I remember also working with mowing scythes, bush axes, dangerously close to sawmill saws, and belts and pulleys on tractors and other farm implements. It is almost unbelievable that none of the children were seriously hurt.

For these reasons, and there are probably more, I believe that it would be naive to think that we could return to this simpler time.

Many people argue today that we are a nation of people with too many entitlements and too many politically correct agendas which must be met. With these entitlements and agendas there would be an outcry for governmental oversight from child protection divisions of local social services, for protection against corporal punishment, auditing of funds to ensure that public moneys were not being spent for religious instruction, and on and on.

But what do we do with those children that society has discarded? What do we do with the homeless child, the emotionally disturbed child? The child with AIDS? The unwashed, unwanted social pariahs? I would hope that you would begin in this conference to address these issues and more.

If anything I have said here today sounds overly harsh or sounds like a criticism of my home, the orphanage, let me make myself clear about some things: I never had to experience violence. I never had to experience crime. I was never abandoned. I never had to choose which parent with whom I would live. I never had to know the shame of being different because I was poor. On the contrary, most of us in the orphanage felt sorry for people we encountered on the outside that we considered poor. I never had to wrestle with "demon rum" or drugs.

Almost to a person, I was surrounded by caring individuals who provided for me and sheltered me from the temptations, pushes, and pulls of society. And I have come to believe that the next best substitute for my biological family was Barium Springs Home For Children. And I will be forever grateful for my home.

BIBLIOGRAPHY

In Re Gault 387 U.S. 1 (1967)
Rothman, David J. The Discovery of The Asylum: Social Order and Disorder in The New Republic. (Boston: Little, Brown and Company) 1971.
Ruffin v. Commonwealth 62 Va. 790, 796 (1871)

BIOGRAPHICAL NOTE

James M. Campbell, MS, is Associate Professor Emeritus of Criminal Justice at East Carolina University. Although retired part-time, he remains active as a teacher and scholar with special interest in juvenile justice, community policy and residential services for children.

It's All the Little Things

How do you know he is better,
  the challenge goes.
  in many little ways I say
  it's all the little things
  that count:
  he no longer runs up the wall
  and across the ceiling
  before coming down again
  to demolish the playhouse.

His tics, although still present,
  no longer race among themselves,
  banging and bumping together,
  like cars at the Indy speedway;
  today he sat in a chair
  and chatted for twenty minutes;
  he wasn't a bag of worms
  nor a ratchet-geared robot.

And now, near friendly people
  peer into the perimeter
  of his monster-inhabited world;
  why, only today from my phone
  he dialed his housemother
  saying, "Where are you Mattie?
  I'm here; come and get me."

That's how I know he's better:
  it's all the little things that count.

Douglas Powers, MD

[Haworth co-indexing entry note]: "It's All the Little Things." Powers, Douglas. Co-published simultaneously in *Residential Treatment for Children & Youth* (The Haworth Press, Inc.) Vol. 17, No. 3, 2000, p. 103; and: *Family-Centered Services in Residential Treatment: New Approaches for Group Care* (ed: John Y. Powell) The Haworth Press, Inc., 2000, p. 103. Single or multiple copies of this article are available for a fee from The Haworth Document Delivery Service [1-800-342-9678, 9:00 a.m. - 5:00 p.m. (EST). E-mail address: getinfo@haworthpressinc.com].

AIDS and a New Generation of Orphans: Is There a Role for Group Care?

Carol Levine, MA

SUMMARY. The AIDS epidemic, now ending its second decade, has created challenges, controversy, and occasionally change. In the early years adults were the primary, and usually the only, focus of attention. Policies and practices affecting children were addressed primarily in relation to HIV-infected infants and young children. Their needs for medical care, foster homes, and nurturing were the focus of specially created private and public programs.

Only in the past several years has the long-term impact of the AIDS epidemic on children and adolescents living with an HIV-infected parent or orphaned as a result of the parent's death come to public and professional attention. Like other aspects of the epidemic, questions about the care and custody of these vulnerable children and youth began to be addressed only after the problem had reached crisis proportions. Also like other aspects of the epidemic, these issues have created challenges, controversy, and occasionally change.

This article introduces one subject that has to date received no sustained analysis: the potential role of group care options for children, youth, and families struggling with the impact of AIDS. This subject has been avoided by both child welfare specialists and AIDS service providers; one barrier to discussion has been history–or to be more precise, oversimplified history. To turn Santayana's well-known dictum on its head, in this case the fear of repeating the past has condemned us to fail to learn from it. *[Article copies available for a fee from The Haworth Document Delivery Service: 1-800-342-9678. E-mail address: getinfo@haworthpressinc.com <Website: http://www.haworthpressinc.com>]*

Carol Levine may be written at United Hospital Fund, 350 Fifth Avenue, 23rd Floor, New York, NY 10118.

[Haworth co-indexing entry note]: "AIDS and a New Generation of Orphans: Is There a Role for Group Care?" Levine, Carol. Co-published simultaneously in *Residential Treatment for Children & Youth* (The Haworth Press, Inc.) Vol. 17, No. 3, 2000, pp. 105-120; and: *Family-Centered Services in Residential Treatment: New Approaches for Group Care* (ed: John Y. Powell) The Haworth Press, Inc., 2000, pp. 105-120. Single or multiple copies of this article are available for a fee from The Haworth Document Delivery Service [1-800-342-9678, 9:00 a.m. - 5:00 p.m. (EST). E-mail address: getinfo@haworthpressinc.com].

105

KEYWORDS. AIDS orphans, new roles for group care, group care for AIDS orphans

HISTORICAL RESPONSES TO DEPENDENT CHILDREN

In discussions of contemporary social policy, appeals to history often take the form of nostalgia about reliving an idyllic past or anxiety about recreating a fearful one. The past is used selectively and rhetorically. This article tries to use a historical perspective in a more balanced and nuanced way: to understand the responses of American society to poor and dependent children, to examine the possibilities for the future, and to identify the impediments and obstacles to achieving just and compassionate social policies.

In colonial America almshouses were established to house poor, disabled, and ailing adults. The first almshouse was created in Boston in 1664. It was designed for those who were incapable of caring for themselves, and who had no relatives who could or would take them in. Almshouse residents included people who were sick, mentally infirm, disabled, crippled, or blind. Widows and orphaned or abandoned children were among them. Younger children stayed in almshouses with their parents, while older children were placed in the community as apprentices or indentured servants. These institutions were intended to provide substitute housing for those who lacked shelter, and for those who for whatever reason could not fit into the community. They were not modeled on the family but were a placement of last resort.

The growth of urban centers in the first half of the nineteenth century and the frequent occurrence of epidemics created even more intense interest in constructing institutions to house orphans and destitute children. The cholera epidemic of 1830 was the motivation behind the creation of some of the first institutions designed especially for children. Typically in the history of such institutions (by the Civil War, some 150 had been built in the U.S.), the impact of epidemics has been overlooked, but both biological and social forces coalesced to spur construction. These institutions typically emphasized the need for discipline and moral indoctrination if children were to be turned into productive citizens (Smith, 1995).

Some children placed in institutions had lost one or both parents, but many had living parents who were unable because of illness or poverty to care for them temporarily or permanently. Some parents paid what they could to the institution for the support. Other children were removed from their homes because of abuse, neglect, poverty, or because the parents were deemed unfit. During what historian Michael Katz (1986) has called the "poorhouse era," the separation of poor children from their parents was pursued as a social goal. The distrust of poor parents was exacerbated by intense fears of social disorder, particularly as waves of immigrants from Central and Eastern Europe entered the U.S.

While orphanages in the early part of the nineteenth century discouraged contacts with living family members, by the second half of the century this isolation began to diminish. By late in the century, a growing skepticism about the harsh discipline and regimentation found in institutions began to inform critiques of the orphanage. Furthermore, the rise of alternative social mechanisms, such as boarding-out (the forerunner of family foster care), adoption, and the growing social antipathy to institutionalization undermined support for the orphanage (Hasci, 1995, 1997).

As an alternative to orphanages, "orphan trains" transported children from cities to farms. Under the auspices of Charles Loring Brace's Children's Aid Society, for example, nearly 100,000 children were moved out of New York City to farm communities in the Midwest and West. Similar programs were created in other Eastern urban centers (Holt, 1992). The impetus was partly moral (to rescue children from the specific vices of their parents and the general moral decay of the city) and partly economic (to provide needed labor to farm families). In some cases, aggressive "reformers" working for groups such as the Society for the Prevention of Cruelty to Children acquired police-like powers to force parents to relinquish their children. Some children found refuge in loving families, after a harrowing process of being exhibited on stages for selection. But the programs were so poorly monitored that there were many instances of physical and sexual abuse as well as exploitation of child labor. Children were frequently separated not only from parents but also from siblings.

By the early twentieth century, with the growth of Progressive reform, serious questions began to be raised about the social and psychological effects of family breakup. The 1909 White House Conference on Children emphasized the need for child "saving" as it recognized the rise in the divorce rate and falling birth rates among white middle-class families. Ultimately these concerns led to the development of mother's pensions in many states. In the 1930s, federally funded support for poor mothers was an essential part of the New Deal, embodied in legislation creating Aid to Dependent Children (ADC) and Aid to Families with Dependent Children (AFDC). This entitlement lasted until 1996, when it was eradicated by the Personal Responsibility and Work Opportunity Act ("welfare reform"). Orphanages that had survived until the 1930s and 1940s fell on hard times economically with the loss of funding to AFDC and foster care and the general disinclination, supported by the growing power of professionals in social work and education, to put children in institutions. Very few continued as institutions to serve dependent children; most either closed or were transformed into residential treatment facilities for severely emotionally disturbed children (Jones, 1989, 1993).

The vast majority of the children who were institutionalized or sent on orphan trains were poor, white, and from immigrant families. A few segregated institutions or sections of institutions were created for "colored" children. For the most part, however, poor, dependent African-American children were cared for by extended families and fictive kin in their own communities. Even where professional services existed, they generally discriminated against minority children (Rosner and Markowitz, 1993).

In the post-World War II era with federal funding, foster care grew rapidly as an alternative to orphanages. Compared to dependent children in earlier decades, foster care systems increasingly had to cope with children who had experienced more severe traumas, particularly through the drug use of their parents or caregivers. Foster care too became overwhelmed by these needy youngsters. As more women entered the labor market and as fewer families felt capable of coping with such troubled youngsters, it became more difficult to recruit foster parents. The child welfare system has been ambivalent toward biological families–at times emphasizing "family preservation" and "reunification" and at times emphasizing removal of children from families for abuse and neglect. As a result, many children never have a permanent or stable home but are moved in and out of foster care, from one foster family to another, from foster family to group home, and then to discharge from anyone's responsibility.

Perhaps the most important lesson to be gleaned from the historical record is the relationship of solutions to the problem of dependent children to the social, political, and economic context of the particular era. There is no clear historical analogue to our own times, no easily adapted model that fits today's children, families, and society (Elder, Modell, and Parke, 1993). Even though they may have served some children well, the historical solutions failed to provide lasting, flexible policies and programs. Instead of looking to the past for solutions for the problems posed by children and youth affected by AIDS, we should be looking for innovative, sensitive, and effective programs that reflect the knowledge gained in the past decades about child development and family dynamics. Even so, there will be no universal answers and no single policy or program that meets the needs of all dependent children.

THE IMPACT OF THE AIDS EPIDEMIC ON CHILDREN AND ADOLESCENTS

The AIDS epidemic in the United States is not a single phenomenon, like the cholera epidemic of the 1830s or the influenza epidemic of 1918. In these cases disease swept through communities, running a more or less predictable course and lasting a definable period. Although illness and death were more common in some population groups than others, disease struck at all social levels and ages. The AIDS epidemic is best understood as a complex series of smaller epidemics, starting at different times in different regions and progressing in different patterns. Because HIV is a bloodborne and sexually transmitted virus, infection occurs among more narrowly defined groups, especially injecting drug users, their sexual partners, and men who have sex with men. HIV can also be transmitted from a pregnant woman to her fetus.

Although AIDS has peaked among the cohort of gay men who were the first to be infected, the incidence of HIV infection is still increasing among women, particularly African-American and Latino women, and among young gay men. At the beginning of the epidemic women comprised about 9 percent of the total; they now comprise 20 percent and in some areas, such as New Jersey, an even higher percentage. Because these women are mostly in their 20s, 30s, and 40s, their dependent children must be cared for during their illness and after their deaths. In some cases the fathers have died of AIDS or are ill; in other cases the women are single parents for a variety of reasons.

In the past few years there have been several encouraging break-throughs in treating AIDS with multidrug regimens and reducing the transmission of HIV from mother to fetus through the administration of zidovudine (AZT) in pregnancy, at delivery, and to the newborn. In 1996, for the first time, death rates due to AIDS declined in New York City, presumably as a result of better and more widely available treatments for opportunistic infections. Death rates for women and minorities, however, have not declined to the same extent as those for white men. Despite reasons for cautious optimism, AIDS will remain a medical, social, and public health problem for the foreseeable future. Even if a cure or vaccine were available to everyone immediately, and no such development is on the horizon, there would still be a long-lasting impact on children, families, and communities.

In 1992 Michaels and Levine estimated that by the year 2000 between 82,000 and 125,000 children and youth (up to the age of 18) would be orphaned, that is, would lose their mothers to the disease (Michaels and Levine, 1992). They predicted that about 30,000 would be in New York City. A subsequent report provided estimates for five other cities: Newark, Miami, San Juan, Los Angeles, and Washington, DC (Levine and Stein, 1994). Although no further national estimates have been undertaken, a 1996 analysis of New York City and State suggests that the earlier figures were substantial underestimates (Michaels and Levine, 1996). This analysis, which included four more years of mortality data from the New York State Department of Health, concluded that by the end of 2001, about 50,000 children and youth (up to the age of 21) would have lost their mothers to AIDS; the statewide estimates reached 58,000. Other estimates have been prepared for Chicago and Illinois and New Jersey.

These numbers are substantial and represent a new and growing phenomenon. In New York, for example, more children and youth are now orphaned by AIDS than by any other single cause; by 2001, there will be more children and youth orphaned by AIDS than all other causes combined.

The scope of the problem is matched by its complexity. While there are many examples of middle-or upper-class families in this situation, the majority of families struggling to deal with HIV illness are poor and from African-American and Latino communities. Even before AIDS, they have struggled with many other economic, social, and medical problems. Drug use by a parent or someone important to the family is the single most influential factor leading to family dissension and dissolution, economic hardship, violence, and inadequate nurturing of children. It has become a truism to say that HIV disease is not the most important issue facing a family at any given moment. Dealing with a parent's illness, however, has a particularly powerful impact on children, even when they do not know (or are not told) that the illness is the stigmatized one of AIDS (Levine, 1993).

POLICY AND PROGRAMMATIC RESPONSES TO FAMILIES AFFECTED BY AIDS

Group care for children and families, the main focus of this article, does not exist in a vacuum. Its strengths and limitations should be analyzed in terms of alternatives that exist or might reasonably be expected to exist. This section outlines the main features of those options. Policy and programmatic responses to the problems faced by HIV-affected children and their families generally fall into four categories: legal changes, funding, services, and housing. In general, programs and policies have focused on stabilizing the family through access to medical, homemaker, drug treatment, and other services; helping the HIV-infected parent make future care and custody arrangements; and providing some social services, such as transitional housing for HIV-infected infants and young children and bereavement counseling for children and caregivers (Draimin, 1995).

Legal Changes. Many–perhaps most–of the children orphaned by AIDS do not have a legalized or even informal custody plan before their parent dies or a legal guardian after a relative or friend takes over their care. Many ill parents do not plan for their children's future, for a variety of cultural, psychological, and practical reasons. One barrier has been existing law. The most significant legal innovation intended to provide a more acceptable process is the establishment of standby guardianship. Seven states (Connecticut, Maryland, Massachusetts, New Hampshire, New Jersey, New York, and North Carolina) now have some form of standby guardianship law. Other states are considering this option. Three other states (California, Florida, and Illinois) have guardianship laws intended to accomplish a similar purpose (Child Welfare League of America, 1997).

Standby guardianship laws originated as an alternative to the unsatisfactory legal options available to seriously ill parents. These were:

name a guardian in a will and hope that the judge awards custody to the named person, or start guardianship proceedings and give up legal rights to one's child. Standby guardianship laws permit a parent with a serious or life-threatening illness to name a future guardian and obtain court approval while he or she is still able to retain custody and make decisions. The standby becomes the legal guardian at the parent's death, incapacity, or other triggering event.

Although there are no data on how these laws are being used, it appears that they work best when there is a readily identifiable and willing standby, when the appointed guardian does not need financial assistance to assume guardianship (since options such as subsidized foster care are closed to legally appointed guardians), and when the family's situation is relatively stable and predictable. Such a fortuitous combination of circumstances is often lacking. Still, the purpose of the law is valid: to give ill parents the power to justify to a court their preferences about future guardians without giving up their rights as parents. The main drawbacks are the lack of appropriate guardians and financial assistance, either a one-time grant for household or other expenses or on a regular basis, to make it possible for poor guardians to take on the economic responsibility for the care of one or more children.

Funding. There is no funding stream currently available that is designed for the special needs of children and youth in HIV-affected families, or to support their new caregivers after the death of the parent. While the parent is alive, many HIV-related benefits such as rent subsidies and homemaker services are available to support her and her family. When the parent dies, these supports and services are cut off. Some funding is available through programs for which the children may be eligible by more general standards; examples are Medicaid, Social Security survivor benefits (if the parent had an employment history); and Veteran's Administration survivor benefits.

The Personal Responsibility and Work Opportunity Reconciliation Act of 1996 ("welfare reform") eliminates federal entitlements to AFDC and gives states block grants to administer programs such as Temporary Assistance to Needy Families (TANF), child care, child support enforcement, food stamps, Medicaid, Social Services Block Grant, Emergency Food Assistance Program, and restrictions on noncitizens. Although the impact will vary according to state implementation, in general it will be much harder for grandparents and other relatives to get public benefits for themselves and for children in their care. Moreover, stringent work requirements will limit the capacity and willingness of family members to take on the care of additional children.

By contrast, federal funds to support foster care, adoption assistance, and other child protection programs were not affected by welfare reform. The result is an economic incentive to put orphaned or dependent children into the foster care system rather than keeping them in their own extended families.

Services. The most prevalent social service response has been the provision of "HIV permanency planning" services. These programs assist HIV-infected parents through the process of determining whether and to whom to disclose their illness, choosing a guardian, negotiating the legal system, and dealing with children's behavior and other problems. Parents are often assisted in creating a "memory book" or videotape as a legacy for their children. Many such programs are organized under the aegis of a larger AIDS service organization, hospital-based clinic, or foster care or child welfare agency; some provide only legal or only social services and coordinate with others for the missing pieces.

Although much publicity has surrounded a few cases in which an ill mother has appealed to the public to find a suitable adoptive parent, in general, relatively few children appear to have been placed for out-of-family adoptions. Some agencies, such as the Council for Adoptable Children in New York, have special programs for placing children whose parent has died of AIDS; and the National Council on Adoption has a campaign geared toward referring potential adoptive and HIV-infected parents to local agencies. Some relatives adopt the children they take in; others reject the idea as unnecessary or inappropriate.

Some bereavement counseling programs have been created especially for children. Some of these programs provide recreational activities such as membership in scouting organizations or experiences in music, art, or drama. Several summer camps have been created especially for HIV-infected children, their parents and siblings. These camps offer one-or two-week stays in a supportive environment. Peer support groups have been organized in a few high schools. Although children's mental health needs are especially important, relatively few services are available that include a complete evaluation and interventions. The Special Needs Clinic at Columbia-Presbyterian Medical Center in New York City is one exception.

Housing. Housing is one of the most significant factors in determining a parent's ability to maintain a stable family and in placing a child after death. Substandard housing, overcrowding, and high rents are the norm in the urban neighborhoods affected by AIDS. Rent subsidies available to people with AIDS have played a major role in keeping a family together through the illness. As noted, these subsidies end on the death of the client. Frequently new caregivers are not able to take over a client's lease and move in with the children. For children, moving after the parent's death is the norm rather than the exception.

Two main types of specialized housing programs have been developed. One is housing created for or available to an HIV-infected parent and her children. These may be in public housing units set aside for this purpose but not otherwise identifiable or in residences specially created for this population. Such programs are in place in several cities, including New York and Baltimore. Services are generally available to assist the family on site or through the sponsoring agency. The second type is transitional housing for HIV-infected babies and young children who do not need to be in hospitals but are awaiting return to their mother or placement in foster homes. The AIDS Resource Foundation in Newark developed such homes in New Jersey; other examples exist in Washington, DC, Richmond, VA, and many other cities. Other non-AIDS programs, such as shelters for homeless youth, are also available in some places.

In sum, a variety of programs have been created, but there is little coordination or continuity. The existing programs serve only a small segment of the population in need. Eligibility is primarily based on the HIV status of the parent; fewer programs focus on children and new caregivers. Families come to the attention of child welfare agencies mainly when there is a crisis and when children may be neglected or abused, but little is available to help them avoid these situations. Finally, the specialized permanency planning and social services were based on an assumption of a "safety net" of federal entitlements that no longer exists, further jeopardizing children's chances for stability and security.

POTENTIAL USES AND BARRIERS TO RESIDENTIAL SERVICES FOR CHILDREN AFFECTED BY AIDS

With the history of historical responses to dependent children as a cautionary background, this section raises the question of whether some new or modified forms of group care would be appropriate to develop to serve families and children affected by AIDS. Such a discussion must recognize the significant attitudinal, managerial, financial, and political barriers that will confront any model program in this domain.

At the same time, it is important to note another inescapable conclusion of the earlier sections of this article: current service models do not meet all the needs of this population, and some children and youth are very poorly served. Some children and youth affected by AIDS may already be in residential treatment centers because of serious emotional problems, which may have been exacerbated but not brought on by the parent's illness. Some are in juvenile justice centers and jails. And some are homeless and live in shelters or temporary housing.

Two assumptions about program development should be made explicit. First, the definition of "family" should be as broad as possible. Family structures in the U.S. are changing, while laws, policies, and services remain wedded to distinctions that are out of date and were probably never applicable in many minority communities. For the purposes of programs servicing children, family members include not only people related by blood or marriage but also people who by their interest and devotion play a significant role in a child's life. Broadening the net to include such individuals makes for some administrative complexities, but it more accurately reflects the resources available to a child. Second, any programs developed for children affected by AIDS must respect community attitudes and norms. Community cooperation is essential to program success, especially for a model that integrates residential care with community-based services.

The focus of this section is on children and families whose difficulties in functioning as a family or in finding a new living situation is closely related to the experience of illness and death. This experience may include prior drug use in the family, domestic violence, losses of other family members, and many of the other social and personal tragedies that pervade poor communities. But without the added stress of AIDS, many families might have functioned reasonably well and many children might have survived by their innate resilience, the support of other adults, or luck. The challenge is to create forms of residential care that address the needs of this group without losing sight of some of the problems that they share with other young people from their communities.

The focus is also on older children and adolescents. Infants and very young children can and should be placed in families–biologic, foster, or adoptive–for long-term care (Berrick et al., 1997). Much of the antipathy toward orphanages results from the inappropriate treatment given to the young children who were the majority of nineteenth-century residents; children over 14 were expected to earn their own living. As the pediatric AIDS epidemic wanes, the transitional housing set up for HIV-infected babies and young children may have to adapt to caring for medically fragile older children, for whom treatment has prolonged life.

There are at least four different groups for whom some form of residential care might be appropriate:

Adolescents Alone. Although data are still scarce, experienced providers report that most children are placed initially with an extended family member, usually a grandmother or maternal aunt. There are no data about the numbers of children who enter foster care immediately after the parent's death or after informal placement in one or more relative's home. Siblings are frequently separated; it is difficult to place more than two children together. Younger children are easier to place than adolescents, who often move from one temporary situation to another or become homeless (Blustein, Levine, and Dubler, 1999).

By all accounts adolescents whose parent is ill or has died of AIDS present the greatest challenge to parents, family members, and service providers. A needs assessment in New York State (Working Committee on HIV, Children, and Families, 1996) asserted: "Planning custodial care for older adolescents is usually more difficult than for young children. From the adolescent's point of view, the assumption of new roles and responsibilities in response to the illness and death of the parent often interferes with their own developmental needs. These issues are risk factors for family dissolution" (p. 21).

A study funded by the New York State AIDS Institute conducted in-depth interviews with 106 adolescents in HIV-infected families. Housing was a serious issue; 28% reported that they had been homeless at some time in their lives, and a quarter feared that they would be homeless in the near future. More than a third did not live with their immediate family. About 40% with siblings see them from time to time, 15% see them only on holidays, and 16% never see them. Nearly a quarter have already been in trouble with the law. Almost all (90%) have been in counseling at some time for bereavement, family conflicts, school and behavior problems, and depression. On their own report, more than a quarter did not read well; nearly 40% reported difficulty in writing; and almost two-thirds had trouble with math. More than half of those 19 and older did not have a high school diploma (p. 21).

Without some significant structure and purpose in their lives, and assistance in dealing with their educational and behavioral difficulties, these adolescents have little hope for the future. A residential setting that provides a safe environment and trained counselors to help these young people make a transition to adult life could be an important model. Residential settings could offer bereaved adolescents the benefits of contact with family without the stress of crowded living conditions and the conflicts inherent in adjusting to a new role living with relatives. Most current group models–group foster care or residential treatment centers–do not address the special needs of youth whose experience includes the illness and death of a parent with AIDS.

The difficulties are formidable: developing peer leadership, ensuring safety and adherence to agreed-upon standards of behavior; resolving conflicts; facilitating contacts with extended family and community; finding jobs or job training; encouraging ongoing relationships with community-based religious and youth and other organizations. And, of course, finding the money and staff to make all this possible.

Adolescent Caregivers. Residential care might also be appropriate for another group of older adolescents, mostly young women: those who have taken on the care of their younger brothers and sisters after the parent's death. Placement of children with an adolescent or young adult sibling is becoming more common; at The Family Center, a service provider in New York City, 15% of custody arrangements now involve an adolescent caregiver. Some of these young women have children of their own. A teenager trying, without assistance, to be mother to her siblings and her own children faces an almost impossible challenge. Residential settings could offer these new caregivers support in parenting, respite from their responsibilities, and companions in the experience. Creating a mixed population of new caregivers with adolescents on their own might offer some synergistic effects in terms of opportunities for social interaction with peers for the caregivers and opportunities for responsible caregiving for the unattached youth.

Children in Crisis. Within the same family children respond differ-

ently to parental illness, and even the same children respond differently as they enter a new developmental phase or react to some external
stress or change. The well-adjusted and cooperative eleven-year-old
becomes a moody, defiant twelve-year-old. The academically gifted
sixth-grader fails in junior high. The thirteen-year-old who willingly
took care of her baby sister turns into a fourteen-year-old preoccupied
with boyfriends. The fifteen-year-old who was her mother's "best
friend" feels displaced by her mother's new boyfriend and instigates
fights with both of them.

In most families and most situations these sorts of transitions occur
without a crisis. But in families dealing with the stress of illness, even
normal developmental changes can result in extreme tension and conflict. The risk is that without appropriate intervention the problem will
escalate. Children with pre-existing conditions such as depression or
learning disabilities are particularly at risk.

At such times a short-term residential placement may give parent
and child, and the other children or family members as well, a safe
space in which to ride out the storm and to deal constructively with the
situation. These are not situations, by and large, in which "treatment"
or a medical model is needed; they are situations in which the normal
stresses of family life are exacerbated beyond the family's ability to
cope because of the additional stress of illness.

Removing the child from constant family tension does not mean
removing the child from the family. Similarly, a parent who agrees to a
child's placement in such a case is not abandoning the child. Rather,
the goal is to resolve the current conflict and find positive ways for
parents and children to communicate and approach future problems.
Joint meetings, activities, and counseling can reinforce strategies for
family functioning. As the parent's illness progresses, there is even
more potential for conflict and tension; timely intervention may help
alleviate some of these strains.

Families Needing Care. There is a significant need to expand the
availability of special housing to accommodate new caregivers and the
children they bring into their lives. Another potential target group might
be a parent reuniting with children after drug treatment or release from
prison; parenting skills could be strengthened in a group residence.
Transition housing, with social services for both children and caregivers, would provide a more coherent way of creating new family relationships and helping sort out new roles and responsibilities.

None of these suggestions remotely resembles the stereotypical orphanage. Even without the distraction of that image, creating new models will require imagination, persistence, and dedication, not to mention money. Bridging the worlds of group care and AIDS care is not an easy task but the potential benefits for children and their families make it an important one.

ACKNOWLEDGMENT

This article is adapted from a report entitled "Staying Together, Living Apart: The AIDS Epidemic and New Perspectives on Group Living for Youth and Families," by Carol Levine, Allan M. Brandt, and James K. Whittaker. The report is based on a October 1996 conference organized by The Orphan Project and funded by the Shelley and Donald Rubin Foundation and the Ittleson Foundation. Copies are available free from The Orphan Project, c/o The United Hospital Fund, 350 Fifth Avenue, 23rd Floor, New York City, NY 10118. The contributions to the project of its co-directors, Allan Brandt, Ph.D., and James Whittaker, Ph.D., and of the participants, are gratefully acknowledged.

REFERENCES

Berreck, Jill D., Richard P. Barth, Barbara Needell, and Melissa Jonson-Reid (1997). "Group Care and Young Children," *Social Service Review*, June, pp. 257-273.

Blustein, Jeffrey, Carol Levine, and Nancy Neveloff Dubler, *The Adolescent Alone: Decision Making in Health Care in the United States.* New York: Cambridge University Press.

Child Welfare League of America (1997). "Newsletter on Standby Guardianship," *HIV Permanency Planning News*, May (Vol. 1).

Draimin, Barbara (1995). "A Second Family? Placement and Custody Decisions," in *Forgotten Children of the AIDS Epidemic*, eds. Shelley Geballe, Janice Gruendel, and Warren Andiman. New Haven: Yale University Press, pp. 125-139.

Hasci, Timothy (1995). "From Indenture to Family Foster Care: A Brief History of Child Placing," *Child Welfare* 74(1), pp. 162-180.

_____ (1997). *Second Home: Orphan Asylums and Poor Families in America.* Cambridge, MA: Harvard University Press.

Holt, Marilyn Irvin (1992). *The Orphan Trains: Placing Out in America.* Lincoln and London: University of Nebraska Press.

Jones, Marshall B. (1989). "Crisis of the American Orphanage, 1931-1940," *Social Service Review*, December, pp. 613-629.

_____ (1993). "Decline of the American Orphanage, 1941-1980," *Social Service Review*, September, pp. 459-480.

Katz, Michael B. (1986). *In the Shadow of the Poorhouse: A Social History of Welfare in America*. New York: Basic Books.

Levine, Carol (1994). "The New Orphans and Grieving in the Time of AIDS," in *AIDS and the New Orphans: Coping with Death*, eds. Barbara Dane and Carol Levine. Westport, CT: Auburn House, pp. 1-11.

Michaels, David, and Carol Levine (1992). "Estimates of the Number of Motherless Youth Orphaned by HIV in the U.S.," *Journal of the American Medical Association*, Vol. 268 (December 23), pp. 3456-3461.

Rosner, David, and Gerald Markowitz (1993). "Race and Foster Care," *Dissent*, Spring, pp. 233-237.

Rothman, David J. (1971). *The Discovery of the Asylum: Social Order and Disorder in the New Republic*. Boston: Little, Brown.

Smith, Eve P. (1995). "Bring Back the Orphanages? What Policymakers of Today Can Learn from the Past," *Child Welfare* 74(1), pp. 115-142.

Working Committee on HIV, Children, and Families (1996). *Families in Crisis*. New York: Federation of Protestant Welfare Agencies.

BIOGRAPHICAL NOTE

Carol Levine joined the United Hospital Fund in New York City in October 1996 where she directs the Families and Health Care Project. She also continues to direct The Orphan Project: Families and Children in the HIV Epidemic, a research and policy development project analyzing the impact of the epidemic on children whose parents are ill with or have died of HIV/AIDS. She founded The Orphan Project in 1991. For 12 years she was on the staff of The Hastings Center. In 1993 she was awarded a MacArthur Foundation Fellowship for her work in AIDS policy and ethics.

"The Giving of Gifts"

Unbeknownst to the other,
each had wrapped a gift
on the last day before
the one for his departure.

On the day of leaving
he handed me a billfold
carefully constructed
through many hours
of secret labor;
it contained a card
with future address
clearly written,
and in capital letters
the admonition:
PLEASE WRITE TO ME.

He noted at once
the empty space
on my crowded wall
that had been occupied by a framed print
that he had always liked
and looked for
on each and every visit.

[Haworth co-indexing entry note]: "The Giving of Gifts." Powers, Douglas. Co-published simultaneously in *Residential Treatment for Children & Youth* (The Haworth Press, Inc.) Vol. 17, No. 3, 2000, pp. 121-122; and: *Family-Centered Services in Residential Treatment: New Approaches for Group Care* (ed: John Y. Powell) The Haworth Press, Inc., 2000, pp. 121-122. Single or multiple copies of this article are available for a fee from The Haworth Document Delivery Service [1-800-342-9678, 9:00 a.m. - 5:00 p.m. (EST). E-mail address: getinfo@haworthpressinc.com].

Before he had time to ask
its whereabouts, I handed him
the package, wrapped,
with address clearly written
and the same admonition:
PLEASE WRITE TO US.

We shook hands and parted,
each changed in ways
both known and unknown
from that day forward.

Douglas Powers, MD

Celebrating Change:
A Schema for Family-Centered
Practice in Residential Settings

Lessie L. Bass, DSW
David A. Dosser, Jr., PhD
John Y. Powell, PhD

SUMMARY. The "schema" (a family-centered, strength-based helping process model) was tested in two (2) children's residential settings. One specialized in longer term treatment-oriented placements, and the other in shorter but more intense and treatment-focused placements. The staff of both programs desired to increase their effectiveness in working with families (or to become more family-centered). The six-step schema (Joining›Discovery›Changing›Celebrating›Separating›Reflection) was intended to guide, enhance, and evaluate family-centered helping processes in both residential settings. A study of its utility was conducted over a one year period. Qualitative and quantitative data were collected to help measure family-centered progress, but an insufficient amount of quantitative data prevented a meaningful statistical analysis. Detailed qualitative interviews, however, yielded data that supported the use of the "schema" as a guide to help promote family-centered practice. *[Article copies available for a fee from The Haworth Document Delivery Service: 1-800-342-9678. E-mail address: getinfo@haworthpressinc.com <Website: http://www.haworthpressinc.com>]*

The authors wish to thank the staff of the Children's Home, Inc. (Winston-Salem, NC) and Nazareth Children's Home (Rockwell, NC) for their thoughtfulness, support and willingness to test the Schema for Family-Centered Practice in their agencies. The Duke Endowment is also thanked for funding the project.

The authors may be written at East Carolina University (Drs. Bass & Powell at Social Work and Dr. Dosser at Marriage & Family Therapy), Greenville, NC 27858.

[Haworth co-indexing entry note]: "Celebrating Change: A Schema for Family-Centered Practice in Residential Settings." Bass, Lessie L, David A. Dosser, Jr., and John Y. Powell. Co-published simultaneously in *Residential Treatment for Children & Youth* (The Haworth Press, Inc.) Vol. 17, No. 3, 2000, pp. 123-137; and: *Family-Centered Services in Residential Treatment: New Approaches for Group Care* (ed: John Y. Powell) The Haworth Press, Inc., 2000, pp. 123-137. Single or multiple copies of this article are available for a fee from The Haworth Document Delivery Service [1-800-342-9678, 9:00 a.m. - 5:00 p.m. (EST). E-mail address: getinfo@haworthpressinc.com].

123

KEYWORDS. Family-centered helping process, guiding family-centered practice, strengths-based practice, family-agency partnerships

INTRODUCTION

Most children spending time in residential settings return to their homes. Family support emerges as a significant factor in determining post-discharge adaptation (Taylor and Alpert, 1973). Thus, it is likely that the future progress of discharged youth and their families will be directly related to the quality and quantity of family-centered services, support, and assistance that they receive during and after placement. Further, using a family-centered helping model that is known to both staff and families should help make residential placement experiences more satisfying and useful for consumers and providers.

Until the development of the "Schema for Family-Centered Practice," social work professional literature contained few "user-friendly," family-centered models to guide practice (Powell, 1996). The term "schema" was taken from the work of Piaget, meaning a mental framework upon which one can organize thoughts and ideas. Traditional practice models (or "helping processes") use disease-process terms (such as "diagnosis," "treatment," etc.). Such terms, while they may be quite useful for physicians and medical personnel treating physical and emotional illnesses, are not compatible with concepts of strengths-based work with family units. Modern family-centered practice is built upon such ideas as (1) developing family strengths, (2) helping families become partners with professionals and helping agencies, (3) using a broad range of community and neighborhood resources to help families, and (4) recognizing that each family has a different and unique culture that can be built upon to help families grow stronger (Fausel, 1998).

As family-centered practice emerged, various approaches and techniques have been suggested. However, many professionals, rather than rigidly following one particular model, have become eclectic in their helping approaches and use a wide array of models and techniques. Recent research suggest that using a particular psychotherapeutic approach makes little difference. Analyses of successful therapy outcome studies suggest that about 30% of successful outcome could be attributed to "therapeutic relationships," 15% to "expectancy, hope, and placebo," 40% to "extra therapeutic factors: clients and their environments," and only 15% to "therapeutic technique" (therapeutic techniques or theories mattered little to clients, but they assisted professionals in organizing their work). But it was pointed out that therapeutic help can be of great assistance to families and individuals especially if professionals emphasize factors that appear to be the most significant such as therapeutic relationships, hope and environmental factors (Miller, Duncan & Hubble, 1997; Hubble, Duncan & Miller, 1999).

Words (terms) are powerful and can convey important messages that can help clients lift their lives to higher levels. The "schema" emphasizes and builds upon the findings of Miller, Duncan & Hubble in several ways: (1) Often professional helpers, while using a variety of family-centered approaches, become confused and lose their sense of direction. The "schema" offers general direction and guidance for therapy, but it also allows for employing a variety of "therapeutic techniques." (2) The "schema" builds upon "expectancy, hope and placebo" by using terms such as "celebration and change." (3) Also, the "schema" enhances "therapeutic relationships" by using terms like "joining," "discovery," "change," and "celebration." (4) Finally the "schema" can be used to emphasize "extra therapeutic factors" such as support from extended family, friends, and formal and informal community groups.

One of the authors (Powell), prior to joining the faculty at East Carolina University in 1987, worked for twenty-four years in residential care agencies. Reflecting upon his residential care experiences, he became convinced that the "schema" could serve as an agency-wide helping process model to guide family-centered practice. Later he was joined by the other authors, and they began to refine the "schema" for use in residential settings. They speculated that rather than having the model known only to professional staff it could be shared and taught to families and professionals from referring agencies. A search of professional literature failed to reveal a model that taught families about or guided families through a helping process. Further, the "schema" appeared to be an easy-to-understand and operationalize generic model that allowed agencies and professionals to employ a wide range of techniques and approaches.

STAFF TRAINING PROCESS

There are six continuous and cumulative steps or phases in the "schema":

1. Joining › 2. Discovery › 3. Changing › 4. Celebration › 5. Separating › 6. Reflection (see Figure 1). The "schema" was designed to help professionals and families experience helping processes differently from tradition pathology-driven models. It is a less pejorative, more optimistic and more hopeful perspective than most previous helping process models. The "schema's" steps or terms (Joining›Discovery›Changing›Celebration›Separating›Reflection) organize practice– not in a lock-step, rigid manner–but by changing basic values that precede process and practice.

The "schema" was first introduced to the staff of the two residential homes for children in Western North Carolina, and it was later field tested in these (2) children's residential settings. One residential center specializes in longer term treatment-oriented placements, and

FIGURE 1. Schema as Continuous Helping Process

Celebrating Change
A Schema for Family Centered Practice

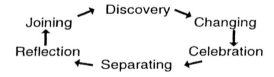

1. **Joining: Engaging families/agency staff.** *Encouraging* families and agency staff to become partners in a process or journey together to meet the goals of the family.
2. **Discovery: Beyond diagnosis.** *Looking* for strengths in families and communities as well as recognizing the reality of their struggles and concerns.
3. **Change: More than treatment.** *Working* together to promote positive changes for children, families, agency staff, and agencies.
4. **Celebration: Recognizing and appreciating strength and potential.** *Attending* to and amplifying change, however small, and affirming growth, potential, competence, confidence and hope.
5. **Separation: Sharing belief in families' capacity to cope.** *Ending* the journey together so that families and agency staff separate; both better for having been on the journey together and with each carrying with them new ways of coping, new possibilities, new life, and new meanings.
6. **Reflection: Opportunity to grow.** *Thinking* through what has happened for both families and agencies and beginning again.

the other shorter but more intense and treatment-focused placements. Two one-day orientation and training sessions were held. Residential personnel from both of the test sites and the authors along with selected trainers met, learned and shared with one another as they discovered and explored the "schema" model. The participants began a "journey" of transforming themselves to use a new model that would later be shared and taught to the families they served and to staff from referring agencies. The "schema" training stressed collaboration and partnership with families (see Figure 2).

A unique feature of the project was that the "schema" would provide family members with the same "process map" that the helpers (residential agency personnel) had and intended to follow. "Schema"

FIGURE 2. Poster of Schema

Celebrating Change

A Schema for Family Centered Practice

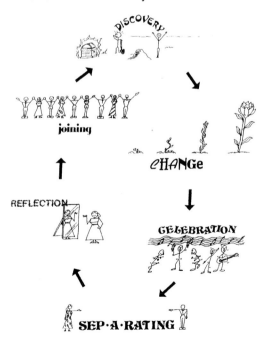

manuals and "schema" pocket cards which had been prepared for use by families were used to train staff. Posters depicting the stages of the "schema" were given to the participants, and later they were posted throughout each residential center.

Historically, helpers have needed theoretical "maps in their heads" to organize and guide their therapeutic efforts. For individual sessions and the entire course of work with the family, helpers believe that the "schema" will assist both consumer and service provider. The "schema" provides the same map for families and professionals so that they can plan and chart the progress of the helping process together.

The "schema" uses deliberate, different, and powerful language that is designed to be optimistic and hopeful. The language is deliberately chosen so that families can understand the stages of the "schema." "Schema" cards can become purposeful as visual aids that provide an image of a helping process and therefore a map for change. The family members received individual "schema" cards at pre-placement conferences. When families are provided cards and given access to what is expected, it is believed that families will accept greater ownership of placements and be more actively engaged in processes of growth and change.

"Schema" family workbooks were developed for families and agency staff to use collaboratively and were distributed to staff trainees. The "schema" was developed as an open, generic model, which allowed the agency staff to use and adapt their "tried and true" methods. The model also challenged staff to think critically, to re-examine and select the most promising approaches. A brief overview of how the six phases were taught to residential agency staff in the two one-day orientation and training sessions is given below. Please note that the training was experientially based with staff member participants "trying out" the "schema" step-by-step, for themselves and offering suggestions which were incorporated into the model and process.

> *Joining:* This step is intended to encourage families and agencies to become "partners" in a process or "journey" together. This journey is in keeping with the concepts of "narrative family therapy" and can be characterized as a "family's story." A musician, songwriter and a storyteller assisted the researchers and residential staff to help create experiential joining exercises. Thus researchers and residential staff joined together in the sche-

ma model to learn how this might be used later with client families.

As staff and trainers "put" themselves into the place of client families by modeling and practicing "joining," questions are raised: *What does joining mean to us, and can we describe joining behaviors that we employ? Exploring natural styles of joining. "How do we join with others? Practicing partnering. How can we, in a limited way, become part of your "family story" as you experience a helping process with us? Developing trust by sharing stories of joy, pain, love and equality. In joining with the residential agency, what has helped to build trust between you, referring agency professionals and the children's home staff? What has slowed down or stopped the "joining" step of the process? What could each of us do to speed up "joining" together?*

After one-half day of joining, the researchers and residential agency staff spent the remainder of the two-day process introducing staff to each step of the "schema" model. Each staff member demonstrated and practiced helping behaviors in each step of the model.

Discovery: In "discovery," an imaginary treasure chest was buried and digging occurs. Using a family story analogy, the discovery step encourages families to think about their family history, traditions, and heritage. The state is set for "This is the reality of what has happened," and it leads to questions like "Now what are you as a family going to do about it?" Residential staff helpers, as a part of their journeys with the families, can help families discover their personal and family strengths and to build upon them. Working to turn disappointments of the past into personal power, how often do we sit down with families and think about discovering treasures? The staff participants believed that the buried chest presented a useful metaphor for discovering and building upon family strengths.

But discovery has another side–facing the reality of the past, accepting the reality of what has happened and most importantly thinking of what to do about changing the present and setting new directions for the future. Questions like, *What is going well? What would you like to change? Let's look at your family history. What are meaningful stories? What strengths, values, and traditions have lasted over generations in your family and that can guide you in the present? What strengths do you have to call on from the past that remain within you, your family system, your friends, your neighborhood and your community? Hopes and dreams for the future can be strengths. What can you call upon from your past family story and from your present life that can help you build a positive future for you, your children, and family?*

Participant awareness included the idea that "discovery" includes using such tools as genograms and eco-maps. Families can learn to use the genogram to transport family history and narrative to the present. Clear genogram instructions were included in the staff's and the family's workbooks. Genograms can assist families to declare positive traditions, retain family sayings, and identify strong past and present family members. Eco-maps encourage families to acknowledge realistic sources of support, energy, areas of stress, stress-free zones, and social support.

Changing: Terms like "treatment" and or "intervention" are generally used, but "change" tends to be less judgmental. While change suggests positive outcome, making changes as an individual or family is not easy. It is a time of hard work. Using the "family story" approach can assist families to begin "writing" more hopeful chapters for their lives. The change process allows families to answer questions related to change. What will it take for change to occur? Who decides if and what changes should occur? Family members (which ones)? Workers? Others? What realistic changes can our family make?

Some ways of thinking about change include: reframing, seeing new possibilities in the life of families, trying on new ways of thinking, weaving "new cloth in an old quilt" and bridging old life histories with new, more hopeful family stories. "Family sculpting" and directions were included in each schema workbook. Changes also need to occur in workers, agencies, policies, resources, attitudes or resources.

Celebration: Powell (1996) noted that celebrations do not need to be ostentatious events at the end of the client/worker relationships, but rather celebrations could be small and quietly observed at strategic points while work is in progress. It is believed that in almost every helping process there will be something to celebrate if we carefully look for and expect positive changes to occur. Thinking about celebration tends to bring out the strengths and potential in families. Celebration can be quiet affirmations of growth, potential, confidence, and hope. It is important to celebrate all changes, even subtle ones.

Celebrating goes far beyond the usual stage of evaluation to help make helping more dynamic and more positive. Celebrating can move the writing of family stories to new levels, as family members experience success and begin to think of positive gains they have attained that can lead to brighter futures for generations yet to come.

Separating: The process of separating was not seen as finishing the joint work undertaken by workers and clients, but rather as a step of "setting families free to carry out their life tasks with greater possibilities of success." In the training sessions, staff recalled separations in their lives and how they tended to "do it the same old way."

As part of a strength based approach, "setting families free to try their own wings" the "schema" step of "separating" opens new possibilities. For example, connecting links can continue between clients and helpers, for example by formal or informal follow-up services. Considering the concept of "separating" is essential as children leave residential care. *Families can carry with them new ways of coping, with new possibilities, new life and new meaning. Separations may leave families with wonderful gifts. What symbolic gifts did staff add to families' story? What did families give symbolically to the cottage or agency?*

Reflection: Opportunity to grow from practice. Reflection is a post-helping step, a time when workers can think through what has happened. Reflection symbolizes renewal and growth for workers, and each act of helping a family. Each act of helping a family, combined with reflection, has the potential of lifting family-centered workers' knowledge, values, and skills to a higher level. Reflection should not occur only at the end of a helping process; it should be a continuous process. Not only do families learn and grow from professional helpers, helpers also learn and grow from interacting with clients.

Reflection represents an opportunity for research and evaluation. In habitually using the reflection process, professionals develop their skills, as is indicated in the schema by an upward spiral of continuous and professional growth.

FINDINGS

After the initial training sessions with the staff of the two participating residential agencies was completed, the "schema" model was used and tested in both settings for approximately one year. The authors (researchers) made field visits to each agency at three month intervals to provide technical assistance and support. Both quantitative and qualitative data were sought, but unfortunately there were insufficient quantitative data for a statistical analysis. However, extensive qualitative interviews were conducted with family members and staff at the conclusion of the study at both test sites. Content analyses of the interviews were made (Lofland, 1971). The results are described below:

H1-Partnership: Does using the schema for family-centered practice in residential care help clients achieve a greater level of involvement, ownership, voice and access?

Qualitative Data Results: Interviews with parents, children, and agency staff confirmed that the schema did help family members and children achieve a greater level of involvement. Representative quotes follow:

> *Yes, I think it's an excellent guide and if it is used the way that you showed us how to use it, I think it will be a successful, interesting . . . to anyone interested in using it.*

> *The only thing I can think of is the fact that parents who we allowed to use the schema; it has helped them as far as being [taking] a role where they don't look for professionals to take charge. They're pretty much at a point where they can take charge for themselves.*

Yes, I think it is a joining process and it also helps to enlighten relationships with staff as well as employees that we come in contact with.

To me, joining is the most important aspect of the whole ordeal. You have to join with the client before you're able to do any of the rest of it. I think there's a way you can come around to join regardless of race, creed, color, whatever you want to call it. And as far as the "stage of change" or did it make a difference in treatment, I feel that it did between the clients that I dealt with.

I think in some ways, too, it helps legitimize my words, you know? If I say, "we want to be in partnership with you" and then can say, "Well here is what we're going to be doing together." I think that helps, maybe, put them more at ease. Again, getting back to them knowing what to expect.

I think it gives families more of a voice and more of a role. The language–it's not technical with things like "assessing" or "diagnosing" and it also helps the counselor and the family understand that they're kind of the experts. They're the ones that have lived with this child for 14 or 15 years. That's something we always tell ourselves, but it's hard to remember that sometimes when you're giving the families advice or working with them. But this enables them to . . . they get to retell their story, and do the exercises, and say "this is what we have done in the past," or "this is what my mother might have done." So I think that's a great way to help them feel like the experts, and help the counselor be reminded of the fact that they are kind of bringing it on the same level.

H2-Focus and Intensity: Does having the "Schema" known and shared by clients and helpers help maintain focus and intensity?

Qualitative Data Results: Interviews indicated that using the schema could help provide focus and intensity to placement processes.

I see it, and I've been able to use it as a way of helping the family, and the counselor understand the process that's getting ready to take place. In residential, families a lot of times come in not really knowing what they're in for. They just want their child to be "fixed," and they don't quite understand how that's going to happen. And I think it can also be helpful to the counselor to understand what is going on. I think it can be used in a large way–in the whole process, or in a small way.

I can think of a couple instances where especially the notebook has given families an opportunity to sit down and do exercises together, which is a rare thing. And I think they gain a lot from those exercises. I think that having a language to be able to understand what they're going through can be a tremendous help because they don't always understand "assessment" or "diagnosis" and "placement goals" or "treatment goals" or that type of thing. So I think that it helps both.

As far as change in my behavior, if anything, I guess it has made me more intentional. Just by virtue of it, of saying, "This is what we're doing together." So I guess, in that way it has changed my behavior–making me more intentional about bringing the family slowly into what to expect.

And then on the personal side of it, I see it as a way for us, the staff, to help joining with the families; helping them feel comfortable with who we are. Helping them know sort of what to expect, which I think puts people at ease, too.

The more you know about what might happen, it takes a little bit of the apprehension out of it. It's a very good visual tool. I think its good to help to have a focus sometimes when you start to wonder "where do we start?" "what do we do?" And that sort of thing.

I think it's a great way to sort of keep yourself in check as a counselor, and as the family. It's a great way to keep focused. It also sort of gives you a guideline. If you realize that you've not quite completed a stage, you can go back or you can go forward, or you can be in two stages at once. And it's great way to figure out where you're at together with the family . . . the family and the counselor and the treatment team or whoever is working.

H3-Satisfaction: Does using the Schema help youth and their families achieve a greater level/sense of satisfaction with services?

Qualitative Data Results: Interviews tended to indicate using the schema helped to create a sense of satisfaction with services.

> *When I see a parent walking through the door and she has her notebook with her, that just reaffirms my belief that families do want, and do believe that changes can take place. I guess it just helps to reaffirm their commitment to the change process.*

> *It's made families more comfortable, and the kids more comfortable. I think a lot of times we deal with, as residence counselors, helping kids be comfortable with the therapy and whatever else goes on. And that's an incredibly intimidating process. A lot of times they don't feel like they have a voice. And I think knowing what is happening helps with that. Knowing that they do have a say in the exercises. I think, in some ways it opens up opportunities to include the children in that process. So I see that as being a great help.*

> *It has changed the way we work with families; I don't know if I've changed my ideas about families. They learn. It's amazing what kids know just by how you operate on a daily basis. And that can be really big when connecting with a kid.*

H4-Greater Appreciation of Self and Family: Does the family story/narrative aspects of the Schema help family members (both adults and children) to have a greater appreciation of their family heritage, ethnicity and culture?

Qualitative Data Results: Interviews did not reveal enough data to confirm or not confirm this hypothesis, but there were some comments suggesting that the Schema might be helpful.

> *There are times when it has helped in getting down to work so to speak because of being able to say, "Oh yeah, let's use a genogram," "let's do the social network map," or something.*

> *I guess the most important thing, family-wise, is to learn the family's story. it is important because that's where you get them to tell their story. You know, as a family tells you their story . . . "we do such and such"; that's a great time to say "Wow, that's*

great. That's obviously something that has managed to work for you."

They've made all these changes, and it's kind of like a new person now and they're having to separate from the ways they used to do things; the types of decisions they used to make; the ways they made decisions.

CONCLUSIONS AND RECOMMENDATIONS

The qualitative data transcriptions of interviews with families and staff strongly suggest that using the schema can help establish and maintain positive family-agency helping relationships during residential placements. After the project was completed, several important questions were raised by a representative of the funding endowment and they were responded to by the authors as follows:

1. *Did the project meet our original objectives?* From our perspective, yes. We conclude from the feedback (qualitative interviews and informal contacts) that the Schema concept can be of great assistance in helping to promote family-centered practice in residential agencies.
2. *What portions of the project were successful and which were not?* Overall it was successful but we became aware of the difficulty in helping staff to maintain fidelity to the model.
3. *What might you do differently if you were beginning this project over?* The above answer (#2) covers the major points for this question, but we would consider using East Carolina University graduate interns to help support and monitor the project. For example, they could meet regularly with the staff and families to help "plot" the progress of the helping process as well as collecting data, a critical point. This would, we believe, increase fidelity to the "schema" model, and enrich the data base.
4. *If the project is continuing, what future plans have been developed and what funding is in place?* An ideal test of the schema would be to have it used as the standard helping process model in a residential agency(ics) over a period of several years.

In summary, the authors feel that the research project demonstrated that a schema-like helping process model has potential to advance family-centered practice in children's residential settings, and they would be pleased to assist other professionals who might wish to experiment with similar approaches.

REFERENCES

Fausel, D.F. (1998) *Collaborative conversations for change: A solution-focused approach to family-centered practice.* Family Preservation Journal, 3(1), 59-74.

Hubble, M.A., Duncan. B.L., & Miller, S.D. (1999) *The heart and soul of change: What works in therapy.* Washington: American Psychological Association.

Lofland, J. (1971) *Analyzing social settings: A guide to qualitative observations and analysis.* Belmont, CA: Wadsworth Publishing Co., Inc.

Miller, S.D., Duncan, B.L., & Hubble, M.A. (1997) *Escape from babel: Toward a unifying language for psychotherapy practice.* New York: W.W. Norton.

Taylor, D.A., & Alpert, S.W. (1973) *Continuity and support following residential treatment.* New York: Child Welfare League of America.

BIOGRAPHICAL NOTES

Dr. Lessie L. Bass is Associate Professor of East Carolina University School of Social Work and Criminal Studies. Her areas of specialty include child and family studies and nurturing programs for parents and their children. Dr. Bass has a passion for permanency work with children and a long history in foster care and adoption.

Dr. David A. Dosser, Jr. is the Director of the Marriage and Family Therapy Program and an Associate Professor of Child Development and Family Relations in the School of Human Environmental Sciences at East Carolina University. Dr. Dosser currently serves as the Chair of the North Carolina Marriage and Family Therapy Licensure Board and is the Past-President of the North Carolina Association for Marriage and Family Therapy. He maintains a practice in systemic therapy at the East Carolina University Family Therapy Clinic.

Dr. John Y. Powell is Professor of Social Work at East Carolina University where he specializes in child and family studies. Prior to his academic appointment he worked for 24 years in residential treatment–including Hillside in Atlanta, GA., and Thompson Children's Home in Charlotte, NC. He serves as Editor of the Book Review Section and on the Editorial Board of this journal.

Index

Adaptation, post-discharge, 124
Adolescents
  adopted, 6
  from HIV-infected families
    as AIDS orphans, 110,116-117
    custodial care for, 116
    as family caregivers, 117
    homelessness of, 114,115,116
    residential care for, 117
Adoption, 6
  of AIDS orphans, 113
Advocacy, for children and their
    families, 4,18
African-American children,
    discrimination toward, 108
African-American families, HIV
    infection within, 110-111
African-American women, HIV
    infection rate in, 109
AIDS (acquired immunodeficiency
    syndrome). *See also* HIV
    (human immunodeficiency
    virus)-infected families
  multidrug treatment of, 110
AIDS orphans, 15,24
  adolescents as, 110,116-117
  adoption of, 113
  bereavement counseling for,
    113,116-117
  bereavement counseling programs
    for, 113
  guardians for, 111-112
  residential care for, 28,117
AIDS Resource Foundation, 114
Aid to Dependent Children (ADC), 108
Aid to Families with Dependent
    Children (AFDC), 108,112
Almshouses, 80,106
Apprenticeships, 80,106

Baltimore, Maryland, housing
    programs for HIV-infected
    families in, 113
Baptist Children's Home of North
    Carolina, xv
Barboff, Rebecca S., 65-76
Barium Springs High School, Barium
    Springs, North Carolina, 96
Barium Springs Home for Children,
    Barium Springs, North
    Carolina, 95-100,101,102
Bellefaire, 22-23
Bereavement counseling, for AIDS
    orphans, 113,116-117
"Bishop Visits, The" (Powers), 63-64
Blackwell, Michael, xv-xvi
Boarding-out, of children, 107
Boys' Town (movie), 19
Boysville of Michigan, 18
Brace, Charles Loring, 107
Brendtro, Larry, 8
  The Other 23 Hours, xiv,16,28-29
Brief intervention models, 24
Bullock, Roger, 22

California, standby guardianship laws
    in, 111
Caregivers, adolescents as, 117
Care managment approach, 87-91
Caring for Troubled Children
    (Whittaker), xiv,29
Carolinas Project, xiv-xv,47-62
  components of
    Core Curriculum Training,
      52,54
    Family-Focused Forums,
      52,53-54

European Scientific Society for
Residential and Foster Care
for Children and Adolescents
(EUSARF) Congress,
plenary presentation, 13-30
Extended family
churches as, 7
residential care as, 8

Families and Health Care Project, 119
Family. *See also* Parents
involvement in residential care
programs, 22,23-24,25
as social support, 23-24,25
Family Center, The, 117
Family-centered practice, in
residential childcare,
xiii-xvii,26
child-centered practice *versus,*
xii-xvii,4-9
components, 124
definition, 49-50
practice principles for, 50
protocol development for, 24
Family group conferencing, 20
Family preservation, 83,108
decreasing emphasis on, 20,56-57
Family reunification, 83,108
in continuum of care, 85-86
mandate for, 81
optimal level of, 86
Family support, 23-24,25
effect on post-discharge adaptation,
124
Florida, standby guardianship laws in,
111
Food stamps, 112
Foster care
in continuum of care, 85
expansion of, 87
funding of, 108,113
increase in percentage of children
in, 19
residential care *versus,* 19,21
Foster parents, burnout of, 85

"Fresh Thinking About Group Care
for Children" symposium,
95

Gelles, Richard, 20
General Accounting Office,
*Residential Care: Some
High-Risk Youth Benefit, But
More Study Needed,* 22
Gingrich, Newt, 19
"Giving of Gifts, The," (Powers),
121-122
Gould, Stephen Jay, 21
Grandparents, as grandchildren's
caregivers, 112-113
Great Depression, 80,98
Group Child Care as a Family Service
(Keith-Lucas and Sanford),
xiii
Guardian Ad Litem program, 53
Guardianship
residential care *versus,* 19
standby, 111-112

Hart, Hastings, 19
Hellinckx, Walter, 14
HIV (human immunodeficiency
virus)-infected families,
105-120
policies and programmatic
responses to, 111-114
funding, 112-113
housing, 114,116,118
services, 113
residential childcare programs for,
114-119
community cooperation in, 115
HIV infection transmission, 109
maternal-fetal, 109,110
HIV permanency planning services,
113,114
Home-based family services, 81
Homelessness, of adolescents,
114,115,116

for client satisfaction, 134-135
for family involvement, 132-133
for maintenance of focus and
    intensity, 133-134
extra-therapeutic factors in, 125
family workbooks for, 128
phases of, 126-132
    celebration, 125,126,127,131
    changing, 125,126,127,130-131,
        135
    discovery, 125,126,127,129-130
    joining, 125,126,127,128-129,
        133
    reflection, 126,127,131-132
    separating, 126,127,131
schema cards for, 127-128
staff training process for, 126-132
terminology of, 125,128,133
therapeutic relationship in, 125
Scholte, E., 14
Sentimentality, toward children, 6-7
Seriously emotionally disturbed (SED)
        children, residential
        placement of, 33-43
Service-centered model, of residential
        childcare, 26
Sharpe, Larry B., 65-76
Shelley and Donald Rubin
        Foundation, 119
Shelters, for homeless youth, 114,115
Siblings, as family caregivers, 117
Smit, M., 14
Social Security, survivor benefits of,
        112
Social services, for HIV-infected
        families, 111,112-114
Social Services Block Grant, 112
Social support, family as, 23-24,25
    effect on post-discharge adaptation,
        124
Society for the Prevention of Cruelty
        to Children, 107
"Space Talk" (Powers), 93
Special populations, family-centered
        practice with, 24-25

Spencer, Sandra, interview with John
        Y. Powell, 33-43
Staff
    team approach of, discussion
        about, xiv-xv,65-76
    training of, 17. *See also* Carolinas
        Project
Staff-child relationship, in residential
        childcare, 16-17
"Staying Together, Living Apart: The
        AIDS Epidemic and New
        Perspectives on Group
        Living for Youth and
        Families" (Levine, Brandt,
        and Whittaker), 119
Stories, 95
Summer camps, for HIV-infected
        children, 113
Supervision, in residential childcare,
        17
Support groups, 39

Team approach, staff discussion about,
        xiv-xv,65-76
Temporary Assistance to Needy
        Families, 112
TFCGCI (Trieschman Family
        Centered Group Care
        Instrument), 50-51,55,58
Therapeutic milieu, 16
Tracy, Spencer, 19
Treatment, specification of, 21
Trieschman, Albert E., *The Other 23
        Hours,* xiv,16,28-29
(Albert E.) Trieschman Center, 49,60n
Trieschman Family Centered Group
        Care Instrument (TFCGCI),
        50-51,55,58

U. S. Constitution, 100-101
U. S. Supreme Court, 100-101
Université Paris, Nanterre, 14
University of Michigan Fresh Air
        Camp, 16